CW01572916

Small Animal Cardiology

The Practical Veterinarian

Small Animal Dentistry
Paul Q. Mitchell, ISBN 0-7506-7321-4

Veterinary Anesthesia
Janyce Cornick-Seahorn, ISBN 0-7506-7227-7

Veterinary Epidemiology
Margaret R. Slater, ISBN 0-7506-7311-7

Veterinary Neurology
Shawn P. Messonnier, ISBN 0-7506-7203-X

Veterinary Oncology
Kevin A. Hahn, ISBN 0-7506-7296-X

Veterinary Parasitology
Lora Rickard Ballweber, ISBN 0-7506-7261-7

Veterinary Toxicology
Joseph Roder, ISBN 0-7506-7240-4

Coming Soon

Small Animal Theriogenology
Margaret V. Root-Kustritz, ISBN 0-7506-7408-3

Small Animal Emergency Medicine
Jennifer Devey and Dennis Crowe, ISBN 0-7506-7370-2

Small Animal Endocrinology
Dave Bruyette, ISBN 0-7506-7420-2

Small Animal Cardiology

O. Lynne Nelson, D.V.M., M.S., D.A.C.V.I.M.

Assistant Professor of Cardiology
Veterinary Clinical Services
Washington State University
Pullman, Washington

Series Editor
Shawn P. Messionnier, D.V.M.
Paws & Claws Animal Hospital
Plano, Texas

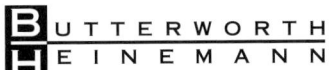

An Imprint of Elsevier Science
Amsterdam   Boston   London   New York   Oxford   Paris
San Diego   San Francisco   Singapore   Sydney   Tokyo

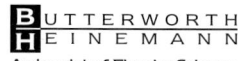

BUTTERWORTH
HEINEMANN
An imprint of Elsevier Science

11830 Westline Industrial Drive
St. Louis, Missouri 63146

SMALL ANIMAL CARDIOLOGY   ISBN 0-7506-7298-6
Copyright © 2003, Elsevier Science (USA). All rights reserved.

NOTICE

Small animal cardiology is an ever-changing field. Standard safety precautions must be followed, but as new research and clinical experience broaden our knowledge, changes in treatment and drug therapy may become necessary or appropriate. Readers are advised to check the most current product information provided by the manufacturer of each drug to be administered to verify the recommended dose, the method and duration of administration, and contraindications. It is the responsibility of the licensed prescriber, relying on experience and knowledge of the patient, to determine dosages and the best treatment for each individual patient. Neither the publisher nor the editor assumes any liability for any injury and/or damage to persons or property arising from this publication.

International Standard Book Number 0-7506-7298-6

Acquisitions Editor: Liz Fathman
Developmental Editor: Kristen Mandava
Project Manager: Joy Moore
Designer: Julia Dummitt

KI/QWK

Printed in the United States of America
Last digit is the print number: 9 8 7 6 5 4 3 2 1

Contents

Series Preface

The Practical Veterinarian series was developed to help veterinary students, veterinarians, and veterinary technicians find answers to common questions quickly. Unlike large textbooks, which are filled with detailed information and meant to serve as reference books, all the books in The Practical Veterinarian series are designed to cut to the heart of the subject matter. Not meant to replace the reference texts, the guides in our series complement the larger books by serving as an introduction to each topic for those learning the subject matter for the first time or as a quick review for those who already have mastered the basics of each subject.

The titles for the books in our series are selected to provide information for the most common subjects one would encounter in veterinary school and veterinary practice. The authors are experienced and established clinicians who can present the subject matter in an easy-to-understand format. This helps both the first-time student of the subject and the seasoned practitioner to assess information often difficult to comprehend.

It is our hope that the books in The Practical Veterinarian series will meet the needs of readers and serve as a constant source of practical and important information. We welcome comments and suggestions that will help us improve future editions of the books in the series.

Shawn P. Messionnier, D.V.M.

Small Animal Cardiology

1

The Heart and Circulation Review

Cardiovascular System Overview

Blood Volume

Total blood volume (TBV) equals 6% to 8% of body weight. Approximately 80% of TBV is located in the systemic veins, right heart, and pulmonary circulation (low pressure system) (Figure 1-1). This low-pressure system has a large capacity and high compliance and is often referred to as a *blood reservoir*.

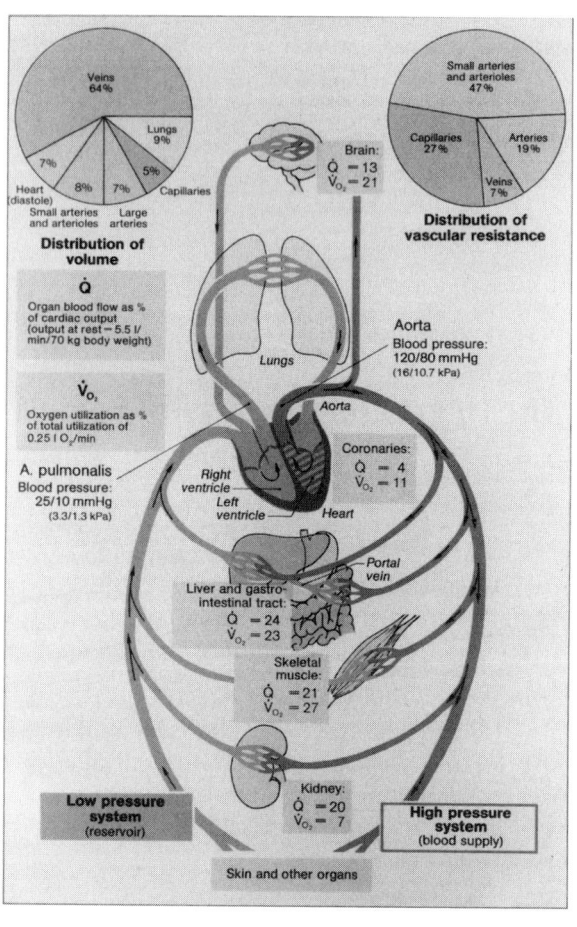

Veins 64%

Lungs 9%

7%
5%

Heart (diastole) 8%   7% Capillaries

Small arteries and arterioles   Large arteries

Distribution of volume

$\dot{Q}$
Organ blood flow as % of cardiac output (output at rest ~ 5.5 l/min/70 kg body weight)

$\dot{V}_{O_2}$
Oxygen utilization as % of total utilization of 0.25 l O_2/min

A. pulmonalis
Blood pressure: 25/10 mmHg (3.3/1.3 kPa)

Small arteries and arterioles 47%

Capillaries 27%   Arteries 19%

Veins 7%

Distribution of vascular resistance

Brain:
$\dot{Q} = 13$
$\dot{V}_{O_2} = 21$

Lungs

Aorta
Blood pressure: 120/80 mmHg (16/10.7 kPa)

Aorta

Right ventricle
Left ventricle

Coronaries:
$\dot{Q} = 4$
$\dot{V}_{O_2} = 11$

Heart

Portal vein

Liver and gastro-intestinal tract:
$\dot{Q} = 24$
$\dot{V}_{O_2} = 23$

Skeletal muscle:
$\dot{Q} = 21$
$\dot{V}_{O_2} = 27$

Kidney:
$\dot{Q} = 20$
$\dot{V}_{O_2} = 7$

Low pressure system (reservoir)

High pressure system (blood supply)

Skin and other organs

Figure 1-1. A summary of the cardiovascular system. This figure demonstrates the major differences between the high pressure atrerial system and the low pressure venous system. Note the contrast between the pulmonary blood pressure and the aortic blood pressure. Also note the distribution of blood volume within the cardiovascular system, the distribution of vascular resistance, and the proportion of organ system blood flow based on percent of cardiac output. *(From Desopoulos A, Sibernagls, eds:* Color atlas of physiology, *ed 4, New York 1991, Thieme Medical Publishing.)*

Cardiac Output

Cardiac output (CO) equals the volume of blood ejected by each ventricle per unit of time. CO equals heart rate (HR) multiplied by the stroke volume (SV). Therefore if HR rises, CO rises. Also, if SV were to fall, HR would reflexively increase to try and maintain CO (common in heart failure). The CO of the left ventricle (LV) is distributed in the systemic circulation to organs connected "in parallel" (e.g., brain, myocardium, intestines, kidneys). The CO of the right ventricle (RV) goes only to the lung (pulmonary circulation).

Organ Blood Flow

The lungs receive blood via two routes: (1) the pulmonary artery conveys blood to the lungs to be oxygenated

(100% of RV output) and (2) the bronchial arteries provide the lung tissue itself with oxygenated blood. Drainage of the lungs is through the pulmonary veins. The brain receives 13% of the cardiac output as its blood flow and is particularly sensitive to decreases in flow and oxygen. The heart at rest receives 4% of the CO. The kidneys receive 20% to 25% of the CO; this is a high percentage in relation to organ size (related to their important regulatory functions). Skeletal muscle and the gastrointestinal (GI) tract both receive about 20% to 25% of the CO. During heavy work, the skeletal muscles may receive as much as two thirds of the CO. The same is true for the GI tract during digestion, but obviously both organs cannot receive maximal flow at the same time.

Blood Vessels and Blood Flow

Systemic Circulation

The blood leaves the left ventricle and flows through the following vessels in this order: aorta, arteries, arterioles, capillaries, venules, veins, cavae, and the right side of the heart. On the way, blood pressure drops from a mean of 100 mmHg in the aorta to 2 to 4 mm Hg in the right atrium. The mean pressure difference (ΔP) and the total peripheral resistance (TPR) in the systemic circulation determine the rate of blood flow (Q), that is, the CO. Thus Ohm's law, $\Delta P = Q \times R$, can apply to the entire systemic circulation or to individual sections in the circulation, such as renal circulation.

Characteristics of Vessels

The velocity of blood flow is inversely proportional to the **common** cross-sectional area of the vessels (fast flow in the aorta/ large arteries → quick delivery, and slow in the capillaries → nutrient exchange). The small arteries and arterioles together account for a vast majority of the arterial cross-sectional area and for about 50% of the total peripheral resistance (a steep drop in blood pressure and flow velocity). These vessels are also referred to as *resistance vessels*. Changes in the arteriolar resistance will considerably affect the total peripheral resistance.

Control of the Circulation

Regulation of Blood Flow

The regulation of the vascular system must ensure that (1) minimum blood flow to all organs is obtained at all times, (2) optimum cardiac activity and blood pressure are maintained, and (3) redistribution of blood to active organs can safely occur at the expense of resting organs. Regulation of blood flow is achieved mainly by alterations in vessel diameter through tension or tone in the vascular musculature (Box 1-1). Vascular tone is affected

Box 1-1. Examples of Vascular Tone Regulation

Autoregulation
Myogenic stretching $\rightarrow$ vasoconstriction
O_2 deficiency $\rightarrow$ vasodilation
Rise in local metabolites $\rightarrow$ vasodilation (e.g., CO_2, H^+,
adenosine, ADP)
Vasoactive substances (kallidin, bradykinin, histamine, AT II)

Neural Control
Sympathetic nerves
Primarily arterioles
Alpha receptors $\rightarrow$ vasoconstriction
Beta$_2$ receptors $\rightarrow$ vasodilation

Hormonal Effect
Adrenal hormones
Epinephrine, low concentration $\rightarrow$ beta$_2$-receptors
Epinephrine, high concentration $\rightarrow$ alpha-receptors
Norepinephrine $\rightarrow$ alpha-receptors

by (1) local effects or autoregulation, (2) neural activity, and (3) hormonal signals.

Arterial Blood Pressure

Systolic blood pressure (SBP) equals the maximum value during cardiac systole. Diastolic blood pressure (DBP) equals the minimum value during cardiac diastole. Pulse pressure (PP) equals SBP minus DBP. Mean blood pressure equals PP/3 plus DBP.

Central Circulatory Control

Central control is effected by the medullopontine regions of the brain. Receptor pathways from the high-pressure system (aorta and carotid artery), the low-pressure system (vena cava and atria), and in the left ventricle terminate in this region. These receptors respond chiefly to stretch. Efferent impulses are then sent to the heart and blood vessels to adjust blood pressure and heart rate.

The Cardiac Cycle

Four Phases

There are four phases of the cardiac cycle, two systolic (I and II) and two diastolic (III and IV) (Figure 1-2). The mechanical events of cardiac action are preceded by electrical events (determined by electrocardiogram [ECG]). Opening and closing of the valves is determined by the pressure on either side of the valve.

PHASE I: CONTRACTION BEGINS All four valves are closed, and the volume of blood in the ventricle remains constant. Pressure rises rapidly. This phase is also referred to as *isovolumic contraction.*

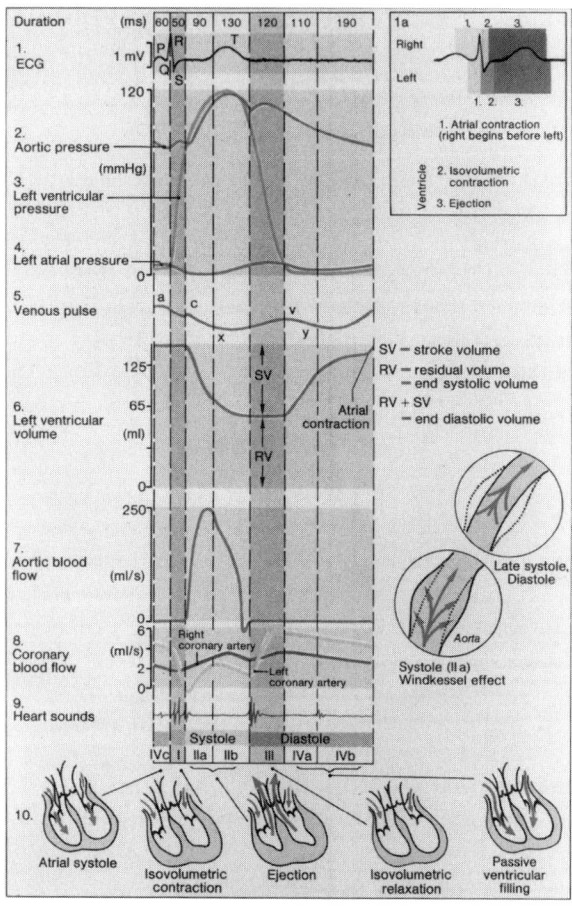

Figure 1-2.   There are four phases of the cardiac cycle. See text for the description of these cycles. This figure demonstrates the findings of various parameters (electrocardiogram [ECG], aortic pressure and flow, left ventricular pressure and volume, left atrial pressure, and heart sounds) during the phases of the cardiac cycle. *(From Desopoulos A, Sibernagls A, eds:* Color atlas of physiology, *ed 4, New York 1991, Thieme Medical Publishers.)*

PHASE II: EJECTION   When the pressure in the LV exceeds that in the aorta, the semilunar valves open. This is the beginning of ejection. Pressure in the LV and the aorta rise to a maximum and then start to fall. When the pressure in the LV declines below the pressure in the aorta, the semilunar valves close.

PHASE III: RELAXATION   After the ejection of blood, the ventricles relax, the volume of blood remains constant, and the pressure declines. This phase is also referred to as *isovolumic relaxation.*

PHASE IV: FILLING   In the meantime, the atria have refilled. When the ventricular pressure during relaxation falls below the atrial pressure, the atrioventricular (AV) valves open and passive filling begins. Active filling occurs when the atria contract, topping off the ventricular volume. The AV valves close at the end of filling as a result of rising ventricular pressure.

Important Points

- Coronary blood flow (myocardial supply) takes place during diastole, especially in the LV, because the vessels are compressed by the contracting muscle in systole.
- Atrial contraction contributes about 15% to ventricular filling normally.
- At higher heart rates, the cardiac cycle becomes shorter at the expense of diastole. Thus atrial contraction and myocardial blood supply become important considerations in tachycardic patients.

Cardiac Excitation and Conduction

Cardiac Muscle

The heart muscle consist of two types of cells: (1) cells that initiate and conduct impulses and (2) cells that conduct but also contract in response to stimuli. The cells that conduct and also contract constitute the working muscle or the myocardium. The ventricles are a functional syncytium, that is, cells are not insulated from one another. An impulse arising in any point leads to the contraction of both chambers. The same is true for the atria.

Conduction Cells

The sinoatrial (SA) node and the conducting system do not have a constant resting potential. The SA node cells slowly depolarize (pacemaker potential) immediately after each repolarization. (The most negative value is called the *maximum diastolic potential.*) The action potential (AP) of the pacemaker cells results from the slowly decreasing outward potassium channel and the relatively rapidly rising inward calcium channels (and some sodium channels). The dominant role of the SA node is due to the fact that the lower portions of the conduction system (e.g., the AV node) have a lower inherent pacemaker frequency than the SA node. Autonomic nervous system (ANS) activity has profound effects on the conduction system. Drugs that alter the ANS (thus, Ca^{2+} and K^+ channels) are sometimes valuable in treating patients with heart disease and heart rhythm disturbances.

Myocardial Cells

In contrast to the SA and AV nodes (fewer sodium channels), the action potential of the myocardial cell is a rapid upstroke from a true resting membrane potential. This rapid rise is due to the brief but fast influx of sodium. The plateau of the AP is caused by the slower-activated inward calcium channels, whereas repolarization occurs due to inactivation of Ca^{2+} and Na^+ channels and increased activity of the outward K^+ channel. These channels are often manipulated with medical therapy, such as diltiazem, lidocaine, and amiodarone, respectively.

Contraction and Relaxation of the Heart

Essential Proteins

The essential components of the heart's contractile apparatus are the proteins involved with contraction (actin and myosin) and those involved with regulatory functions (troponin and tropomyosin). A very small proportion of the myofibril (~10%) is concerned solely with structural proteins (e.g., C proteins, M-line).

Molecular Events

ATP and calcium must be present for contraction. Myosin ATPase splits ATP in amounts sufficient for contraction when it interacts with actin. This interaction is controlled by the regulatory proteins troponin and tropomyosin in a calcium-dependent manner. In diastole, the interaction between actin and myosin is suppressed because of the inhibitory effect of troponin. When calcium is supplied, the inhibitory effect is overcome, and actin and myosin form crossbridges. As the calcium concentration rises, more cross-bridges are recruited and more tension develops for contraction. Relaxation occurs as cross-bridge activity diminishes in response to a falling calcium concentration. Beta-receptor stimulation by catecholamines causes increased cytosolic calcium and allows more cross-bridges to interact, creating stronger tension and contraction. Beta-receptor blockers are sometimes used to decrease the force of contraction and slow heart rate in patients with myocardial hypertrophy.

Frank-Starling Law

If all other factors are equal, the greater the volume of blood in the ventricle just before it contracts (preload), the more vigorous is the force of contraction. This occurs because stretching of the myofibril sensitizes the contractile proteins to the prevailing calcium concentration, causing increased cross-bridge interactions and greater tension generation.

2

The Cardiovascular Examination

Signalment and History

Young animals usually present with congenital disease (i.e., subaortic stenosis), whereas older animals typically present with acquired diseases (i.e., degenerative valve disease or neoplasia). Some congenital heart defects are more common in certain breeds of dogs and cats, and the same is also true for some acquired diseases. The gender of the patient can also be important information because specific diseases can be more commonly seen in male versus female patients.

Important Historical Information

Obtaining an appropriate history can help a clinician determine chronicity and severity, as well as provide important clues regarding etiology of the symptoms. Likewise, understanding what medications are being administered (and patient response) can help confirm suspected disease processes and be crucial in assessing changes in therapy and doses. Box 2-1 contains useful historical information that may be obtained from the pet's owner.

Box 2-1. Commonly Obtained Historical Information

1. Presenting complaint, onset, duration, and progression?
2. Where was the pet obtained?
3. Vaccination history?
4. Where is the animal housed, how closely is the pet supervised?
5. What is the general attitude?
6. Has the pet's activity level changed?
7. Is the pet coughing? Frequency? Character?
8. Is there heavy breathing or excessive panting?
9. Have there been any episodes of weakness or collapsing?
10. What is the normal diet?
11. Any changes in appetite?
12. Has there been any vomiting or diarrhea?
13. Any change in urinary habits?
14. What medications are being administered? When? How much? Response?

Cardiac Versus Respiratory Cough

Coughing may be a symptom of heart or respiratory disease. Some patients may be affected with both disorders. It can be challenging for the clinician to differentiate between cardiac and respiratory coughing. Table 2-1 provides clues to aid in differentiating cardiac versus respiratory causes of cough. In most cases, a thorough history, physical examination with auscultation, and chest radiographs determine the cause of the cough. Occasionally, other tests may be needed.

Observation

Evaluation of the patient should always begin with general observation before physical examination. Pertinent observations should include attitude, level of anxiety, body condition, fluid accumulations (e.g., peripheral edema or ascites), posture, and especially, respiratory rate and character. Important clues regarding the patient's condition may be altered by handling (e.g., pet's excitement may mask significant depression or lethargy, and its respiratory rate may be falsely elevated) if careful observation is omitted.

Table 2-1.   Clues to Aid in Differentiating Cardiac Versus Respiratory Causes of Cough

	Suggests Cardiac	Suggests Respiratory
History	Cough with exercise or excitement Soft cough with tachypnea Decrease in activity Weight loss or inappetence	Cough with exercise/excitement Loud or honking cough +/– terminal gag No activity change No weight loss
Physical examination and auscultation	Tachypnea/dyspnea Crackles (end-inspiratory and expiratory) Murmur	+/– Tachypnea +/– Crackles (inspiratory) or normal lung sounds +/– Murmur
ECG	Sinus tachycardia, arrhythmias +/– p mitrale	Pronounced respiratory arrhythmia +/– p pulmonale
Thoracic radiographs	Cardiac enlargement (i.e., left atrium) Interstitial edema Normal cytology	+/– Cardiac enlargement Bronchial infiltrate Airway collapse
Bronchial wash	Diuretic responsive	Inflammatory or other infiltrate
Medical therapy		Incomplete to nonresponsive to diuretics

Examination

Mucous Membranes

Mucous membrane color and capillary refill time are used to estimate the patient's peripheral perfusion. Capillary refill time (CRT) is assessed by applying enough digital pressure to blanch a membrane; color should return within 2 seconds. Oral membranes (most commonly), prepuce or vagina membranes, and ocular conjunctivae can be assessed for color. In many cases, it may be advantageous to assess mucous membranes in multiple locations (e.g., differential cyanosis of reversed patent ductus arteriosus [PDA]). Box 2-2 lists differentials for mucous membrane color.

Box 2-2. Differentials for Mucous Membrane Color

Pale: anemia, peripheral vasoconstriction
Bright red: excitement, peripheral vasodilation, sepsis, polycythemia
Blue/gray: airway disease, pulmonary parenchymal disease, right-to-left cardiac shunt, hypoventilation, shock, methemoglobinemia
Icteric: hemolysis, hepatobiliary disease

Jugular Veins

Examination of the jugular veins reveals information about right heart filling pressures. The jugular veins should be examined when the patient is standing in a natural position, with the nose parallel to the floor. Ethyl alcohol may be used to dampen the hair overlying the vein for better visualization. Shaving a small spot on the neck may be necessary in some thick-coated animals. Jugular pulse waves are related to right atrial (RA) contraction and filling.

Box 2-3 lists causes of jugular pulsations and jugular distension.

Box 2-3.   Causes of Jugular Pulsations and Jugular Distension

---

Jugular Pulsations
Tricuspid insufficiency
Hypertrophied or noncompliant right ventricle (e.g., pulmonic stenosis, pulmonary hypertension)
Certain arrhythmias (e.g., complete heart block)

Jugular Distension (+/– pulsations)
Occlusion of the cranial vena cava or right atrium by external compression, mass, or thrombosis
High right heart filling pressures (e.g., chronic congestive failure, pericardial effusion)

HEPATOJUGULAR REFLUX Impaired right heart filling can be evaluated using a reflux test. With the animal standing in a natural position, firm pressure is applied to the cranial abdomen (temporarily increasing venous return to the right side of the heart). The jugular veins are examined. Normal animals should have little to no change in the jugular vein. Jugular distension and pulsation that persists during the compression constitutes an abnormal test (impaired right heart filling).

PSEUDOJUGULAR PULSATION Carotid arterial pulses can sometimes mimic a jugular pulse especially in thin or excited patients. To differentiate, apply light pressure to the area of the pulsation. The arterial pulse will continue; the jugular pulse will stop.

Precordium

The precordium is evaluated by placing each hand on each side of the patient's chest wall over the region of the heart (palpable heartbeat). Normally, the strongest impulse is felt during systole on the left side (left apex) between the fourth and sixth intercostal spaces. Shifting of the precordial impulse or decreased intensity may alert the clinician to possible pathology (Box 2-4).

PRECORDIAL THRILL Some animals with loud murmurs have a palpable buzzing sensation on the chest wall over

Box 2-4.   Causes of Shifted Precordial Impulse and
Decreased Intensity of Precordial Impulse

Causes of Shifted Precordial Impulse
Cardiac enlargement (e.g., right heart hypertrophy → prominent
right precordium)
Mass lesions displacing the heart
Collapsed lung lobes allowing cardiac displacement
Focal accumulations of air or fluid

Causes of Decreased Intensity of Precordial Impulse
Obesity
Pleural effusion
Pericardial effusion
Weak cardiac contractions
Thoracic masses
Pneumothorax

---

the heart (palpable murmur) called the *precordial thrill.*
The vibrations are usually felt over the point of maximal
intensity (PMI) of the murmur.

PERCUSSION   Lightly "thumping" the patient with a fin-
ger may help determine the presence of masses or fluid
lines, especially in the thorax. A hollow sound should
normally be elicited over the lungs. A dull sound is
noted over solid structures and fluids.

Abdomen

The abdomen should be evaluated in all cardiac patients. It should be inspected for ascites and hepatosplenomegaly (signs of right heart failure) and evaluated for the presence of masses (sometimes related to cardiac disease, i.e., hemangiosarcoma).

Femoral Pulses

The strength, regularity, and pulse rate are assessed by palpating a peripheral artery, usually the femoral artery. The evaluation of pulse strength is somewhat subjective and requires experience and practice. Femoral arterial pulses can be difficult to appreciate in cats, even when they are normal. Both femoral arteries should be evaluated simultaneously and compared. A weaker or absent pulse on one side may indicate a serious problem such as thromboembolism. The pulse strength is based on the difference between systolic and diastolic arterial pressures (pulse pressure). When the difference is wide, the pulse feels strong, and vice versa.

HYPERKINETIC PULSES Pulses that feel more prominent than normal are termed hyperkinetic. Common causes include high adrenergic tone, PDA, and aortic regurgitation.

HYPOKINECTIC PULSES Pulses that feel weaker than normal are caused by reduced stroke volume. This can occur with heart failure, hypovolemia, and some arrhythmias.

PULSE DEFICIT Fewer femoral pulses than palpable or auscultable heartbeats usually indicates an arrhythmia. An electrocardiogram (ECG) should be evaluated when pulse deficits are found in a patient.

Auscultation

Auscultation is useful to identify normal and abnormal heart sounds, assess heart rhythm and rate, and evaluate lung sounds. Heart sounds are created by turbulent blood flow (e.g., high-velocity flow, incompetent valves, shunts) and by vibrations of the heart and vessels (e.g., normal sounds, gallops). Heart sounds can be described as transient sounds (short duration) (Table 2-2) or murmurs (longer sounds occurring during normally quiet periods).

Murmurs

Cardiac murmurs are described based on timing within the cardiac cycle, intensity, point of maximal intensity (PMI), radiation over the chest wall, and quality and pitch.

Table 2-2. Transient Heart Sounds

Transient Heart Sound	Etiology	Pathologic Condition
S_1	The first heart sound is a normal sound caused by closure of the atrioventricular valves and vibrations of the cardiac walls with abrupt deceleration of blood flow. S_1 is typically longer and lower pitched than the second heart sound	A *split S_1* can be heard with conduction alterations (right bundle branch, ventricular premature contractions), or it can be normal in large dogs.
S_2	The second heart sound is produced by closure of the semilunar valves. It is heard loudest over the aortic area.	A *split S_2* can occur due to delayed closure of the pulmonic valve (pulmonary hypertension, right bundle branch block, ventricular premature beats, pulmonic stenosis, etc.) or due to paradoxical delayed closure or the aortic valve (left bundle branch block, ventricular premature contractions, subaortic stenosis, systemic hypertension, left ventricular failure).
S_3	The third heart sound is due to vibrations in the heart walls associated with rapid ventricular filling. It is a normal sound in large animals such as horses.	In dogs and cats, an S_3 is associated with dilated cardiomyopathy and is referred to as an *S_3 gallop*.
S_4	The fourth heart sound is caused by atrial contraction. It is also normally heard in large animals.	An S_4 can be auscultated in dogs and cats when the atria dilate in response to ventricular stiffness such as in hypertrophic cardiomyopathy (*S_4 gallop*).
Systolic click	A transient click can sometimes be heard in mid-to-late systole over the mitral valve. This is usually the result of delayed closure or tensing of a portion of the mitral valve.	Systolic clicks typically related to mitral valve abnormalities (i.e., endocardiosis). They can occasionally be found over the tricuspid valve.

TIMING WITHIN THE CARDIAC CYCLE *Systolic murmurs* can occur at any point between S_1 and S_2. Protosystolic (early, just after S_1), mesosystolic (midsystole), telesystolic (late, just before S_2), and holosystolic (throughout systole) are commonly used terms. *Diastolic murmurs* are usually heard early in diastole (just after S_2) or throughout diastole. *Continuous murmurs* occur throughout systole and diastole (no quiet period) (Figure 2-1).

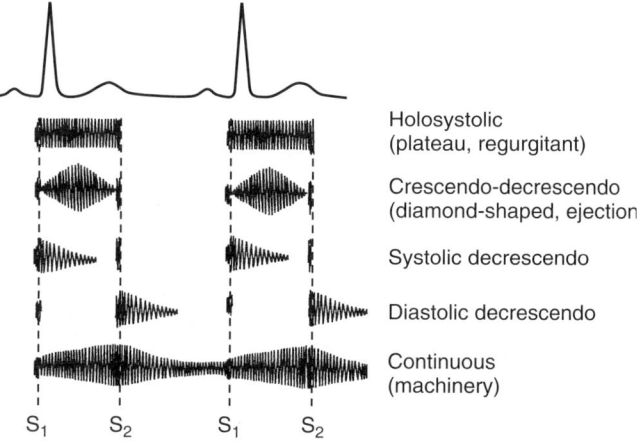

Holosystolic
(plateau, regurgitant)

Crescendo-decrescendo
(diamond-shaped, ejection

Systolic decrescendo

Diastolic decrescendo

Continuous
(machinery)

S_1 S_2 S_1 S_2

Figure 2-1. Approximate locations of various valve areas on chest wall. *T*, Tricuspid; *P*, pulmonic; *A*, aortic; *M*, mitral. *(From Ware WA: Approximate locations, murmur shapes, and neuronohmonal mechanisms. In Nelson RW, Couto CG, eds: Small animal internal medicine, ed 2, St Louis, 1998, Mosby.)*

INTENSITY The intensity of a murmur is arbitrarily graded on a scale of I to VI. This system is used to characterize the murmur, but *it is not used to assess severity of disease.*

Grade I: A very soft, focal murmur detected after several minutes of listening.

Grade II: A soft murmur, readily ausculted and localized.

Grade III: A moderate intensity murmur, ausculted in more than one location.

Grade IV: A moderate-to-loud murmur, radiating well over the chest wall, no palpable thrill.

Grade V: A loud murmur, radiates well, accompanied by a palpable thrill.

Grade VI: Grade V plus audible when the stethoscope is removed from the chest wall.

POINT OF MAXIMAL INTENSITY The PMI is usually described by the hemithorax, valve area, or base or apex location where the murmur is the loudest (Figure 2-2). For example, the loudest point ausculted in the left apical region or left hemithorax over the 4th intercostal space at the costochondral junction would be the typical PMI description for mitral regurgitation.

RADIATION OVER THE CHEST WALL A murmur may radiate from the PMI to other cardiac regions and even noncardiac regions such as the thoracic inlet and calvarium (i.e., subaortic stenosis).

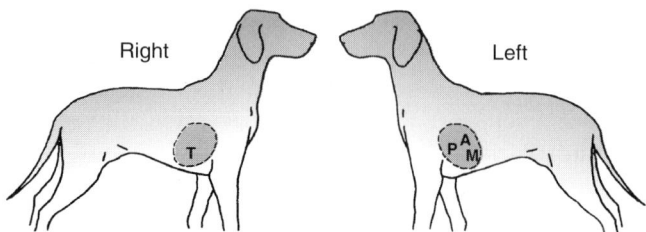

Figure 2-2. Murmur shapes and descriptions, Phonocardiographic shapes and timing, of different murmurs are depicted and described. *(From ware WA: Approximate locations, murumur shapes, and neuronormonal mechanisms. In Nelson RW, Couto CG, eds: Small animal internal in medicine, ed 2, St Louis, 1998, Mosby.)*

QUALITY AND PITCH Murmurs can also be described according to their quality, frequency, and characteristic shape (change in intensity throughout the cycle) recorded by a phonocardiogram (see Figure 2-1). High-frequency sounds may be described as musical, whereas mixed frequency sounds are often described as harsher ejection quality.

Respiratory Sounds

NORMAL SOUNDS Bronchial sounds are normal sounds and are created by air moving through the larger airways and trachea. They are considered tubular sounds, that is, air moving through a hollow tube. Vesicular sounds are normal airway sounds that are created by air moving through the small airways. The sounds are soft and breezy, and have been likened to wind rustling through fall leaves on a tree. They are best heard in peripheral lung regions. Bronchovesicular sounds are a combination of the two and are best heard over the perihilar region, where the transition of large to small airways may occur.

ABNORMAL SOUNDS   *Attenuated bronchovesicular sounds* may be secondary to obesity, pleural effusion, shallow respirations, consolidated lung parenchyma, pneumothorax, or thoracic masses. *Crackles* are nonmusical discontinuous sounds that have been likened to sound made when crumpling paper. They are usually associated with fluid or exudate in the interstium and small airways. They may be inspiratory or expiratory or both, depending on the disease state. *Wheezes* are musical, high-pitched continuous sounds, which suggest airway narrowing. Typically they are inspiratory sounds. *Stertor* and *stridor* are discontinuous sounds (gurgles and wheezes) that are heard without a stethoscope. They are indicative of upper large airway disorders.

3

Diagnostic Methods for the Cardiovascular System

Radiology

Thoracic radiography is helpful in localizing a problem in an organ system in patients with respiratory symptoms, that is, symptoms of cardiac, pulmonary airway, pleural space, or mediastinal disease. In patients with suspected cardiac disease, radiographs are important to assess changes in heart shape and size, as well as to assess the presence or absence of heart failure. Evaluation of intrathoracic blood vessels can also give important clues regarding cardiac disease. Chest conformation must be considered in dogs when evaluating thoracic films. Prominent barrel-shaped chest or deep chest breeds may have a significantly different appearance of the normal heart and thoracic cavity.

Cardiomegaly

Cardiac enlargement may be generalized or localized to a side or chamber, such as left-sided cardiomegaly or left atrial enlargement. Most heart disorders that cause eccentric or concentric hypertrophy affect at least two chambers, that is, tricuspid valve dysplasia with regurgitation causes right ventricular and right atrial enlargement. Generalized cardiomegaly can usually be differentiated from cardiomegaly caused by pericardial effusion by the presence of normal heart contours. Distension of the pericardial sac with fluid, blood, or viscera tends to create a smooth, globoid cardiac appearance on radiographs. Table 3-1 shows commonly used references for cardiac size assessed from the thoracic radiograph. Figure 3-1 shows common radiographic enlargement patterns.

Intrathoracic Blood Vessels

Pulmonary vessels may appear generally prominent or overcirculated (ventricular septal defect, patent ductus arteriosus) or undercirculated (severe pulmonic

Table 3-1. Commonly Used References for Cardiac Size from the Thoracic Radiograph

Species Versus Radiographic View	Lateral Projection	Dorsoventral Projection
Dog	*Height:* Cardiac base ≤two thirds the size of the chest cavity height (apex-spine dimension)	*Length:* ≤5 intercostal spaces
	Width: ≤2.5–3.5 intercostal spaces	*Width:* maximal width ≤two thirds of the width of chest cavity at same level
Cat	*Height:* similar to dog	*Length:* similar to dog
	Width: similar to dog, cardiac apex should not overlap with diaphragm	*Width:* maximal width ≤half the width of chest cavity at same level

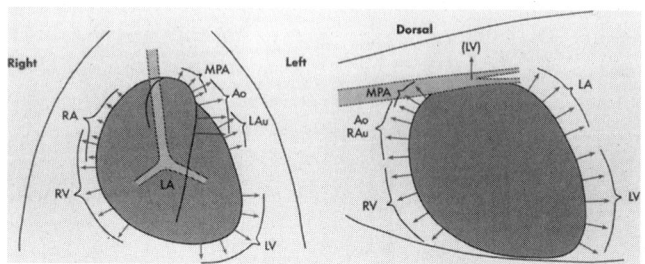

Figure 3-1. Common radiographic enlargement patterns. (*From Bonagura JD, Beckwith L: Common radiographic enlargement patterns. In Fenner WR, ed:* Quick reference to vertinary medicine, *ed 3, Philadelphia, 2000, Lippoincott, Williams & Wilkins.*)

stenosis). *Pulmonary arteries* appear larger than the accompanying pulmonary vein in cases of pulmonary arterial hypertension (PAH). Often, terminal portions of the arteries are attenuated. Causes of PAH may include chronic pulmonary parenchymal disease, chronic airway obstruction, Einsenminger's complex, and heartworm disease. In heartworm disease, the pulmonary arteries may become markedly tortuous. Pulmonary venous hypertension (i.e., left-sided heart failure) may manifest as engorged *pulmonary veins* relative to the arteries. The *caudal vena cava* may be enlarged in cases of systemic venous hypertension (i.e., right-sided heart failure). Other abnormalities in vessel conformation may occur in certain congenital anomalies. Patent ductus arteriosus causes a dilation of the descending portion of the aorta (turbulence adjacent to the ductus) noted on the dorsoventral (DV) radiographic view. This is referred to as a *ductus bump*. Dilation of the main pulmonary artery *(post-stenotic dilation)* caused by pulmonic stenosis is often seen on the DV radiograph in the 1 o'clock to 2 o'clock position. Subaortic stenosis can also cause a post-stenotic dilation of the ascending aorta typically noted as a bulge in the cranial heart base region on the lateral radiograph.

Pulmonary Edema

Cardiogenic pulmonary edema is fluid accumulating in the lung interstitium by "leaking" pulmonary capillaries because of an increase in hydrostatic pressure, that is, left-sided congestive heart failure. An interstitial pattern is usually described as an increase in opacity to the parenchymal tissues with a loss of vessel definition. The opacities may have a hazy and patchy appearance. An alveolar pattern may be noted when fluid moves from the interstitial space into the alveoli. The fluid-filled alveoli become silhouetted against the airways they surround (air bronchogram). In the dog, cardiogenic edema commonly is distributed symmetrically in the perihilar and dorsal lung fields. Pulmonary edema in cats is often patchy and may be focal or unevenly distributed.

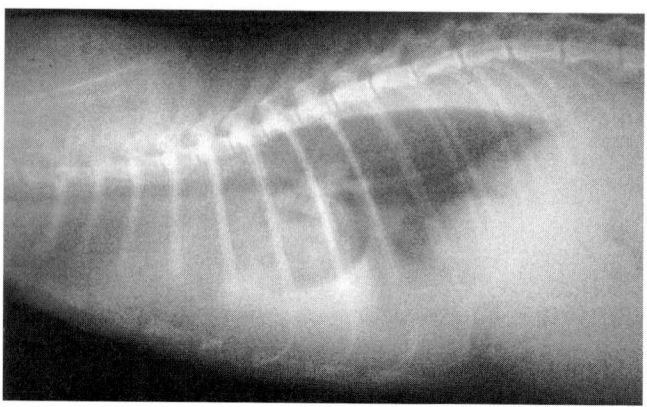

Figure 3-2.   This lateral thoracic radiograph in a feline patient displays typical features of pleural effusion, generalized increase in opacity (particularly ventrally), scalloped ventral lung margins, and lobar retraction from the chest wall.

Pleural Effusion

Fluid in the pleural space typically causes an overall increase in thoracic opacity and obliteration of the cardiac silhouette (especially in the DV projection). Interlobar pleural fissures and separation of the visceral pleural margin form the chest wall are usually noted. Commonly, the ventral lung margins appear scalloped as the lung "floats" on the fluid line (Figure 3-2).

Electrocardiography

The electrocardiogram (ECG or EKG) is an evaluation of the heart's electrical activity (depolarization and repolarization) as assessed from the body surface. The normal heart rhythm (sinus rhythm) originates in the sinoatrial node of the right atrium and is conducted through the atria, atrioventricular node, His bundle, Purkinje fibers, and finally, the ventricular muscle tissue. Each waveform (P, PR interval, QRS, QT interval, and T) generated gives regional information on depolarization or repolarization and conduction in the heart. Table 3-2 gives the normal measurements for the canine and feline ECG.

Indications to Obtain an Electrocardiogram

- To diagnose an arrhythmia detected on physical examination.
- To search for an arrhythmic cause of syncope or episodic weakness.
- To assess cardiac chamber size (a normal ECG does not exclude cardiomegaly).
- To monitor a critical patient (i.e., after hit by car [HBC] trauma or gastric dilatation volvulus [GDV] syndrome).
- To individualize therapy for heart patients (monitor rate and rhythm).
- To evaluate patient with suspected drug toxicosis (digoxin, procainamide).

Table 3-2.   Normal Measurements for the Canine and Feline ECG[†]

Parameter	Dogs	Cats
Heart rate	70–160 bpm*	150–220
P wave (max)	0.04 sec and 0.4 mV	0.04 sec and 0.2 mV
PQ interval	0.06–0.13 sec	0.05–0.09 sec
QRS (width)	0.04–0.05 sec	0.04 sec
R wave (max)	Up to 3 mv (3.5 giant breed or sighthound)	Up to 0.9 mv, QRS total <1.2 mV
ST segment	Within 0.2 mV from baseline	No change from baseline
T wave	Not > 1/3 R wave	0.3 mV maximum
QT interval	0.15–0.25 sec	0.12–0.18 sec
Electrical axis (frontal plane)	40–100 degrees	0–160 degrees

*Slower heart rates are typically noted for larger breeds of dogs, whereas faster heart rates are common in small breeds.

[†]All measurements are evaluated on the Lead II tracing at 50 mm/sec paper speed.

- To screen for electrolyte abnormalities (i.e., hyperkalemia).
- To look for supportive evidence of other disease processes (i.e., low voltage complexes and electrical alternans with pericardial effusion)

What the ECG Does Not Determine

- Strength of myocardial contraction
- Presence or absence of heart failure
- If a patient will survive an anesthetic episode

Electrocardiogram Waveforms

Each waveform (P, PR interval, QRS, QT interval, and T) generated gives regional information on depolarization or repolarization and conduction. Complexes are assessed in Lead II at 50 mm/sec paper speed.

The P wave results from atrial depolarization. The PR (PQ) interval reflects time taken for the impulse to conduct from the SA node, through the AV node and to the ventricles. The measurement is done from the beginning of the P wave to the beginning of the Q wave. The QRS complex results from ventricular depolarization. By definition, the Q wave is the first negative deflection after the P wave and represents depolarization of the septum. The R wave is the first positive deflection after the P wave and represents depolarization of the ventricles. The S wave is the first negative deflection after the

R wave and represents depolarization of the basilar ventricular walls. The T wave results from ventricular repolarization. T waves can be positive, negative, or biphasic, but they should not change polarity on serial ECGs. Large T waves can be seen with myocardial hypoxia, interventricular conduction disturbance, bradycardia, ventricular enlargement, and hyperkalemia. The QT interval indicates the duration of ventricular systole. See Figure 3-3 for the proper measurement of the P-QRS-T complex, and Table 3-3 for a summary of alterations in P-QRS-T wave morphology.

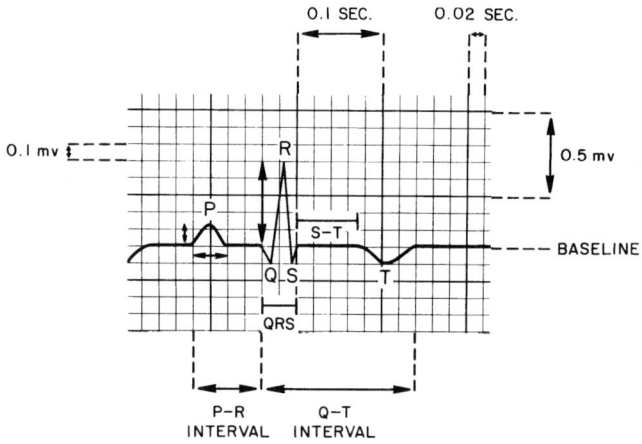

Figure 3-3. The appropriate manner to measure the P-QRS-T complex. (*From Tilley LE:* Essentials of canine and feline electrocardiography, *ed 3, 1992, Lea & Febiger.*)

Table 3-3. Summary of Alterations in P-QRS-T Wave Morphology

Waveform Alteration	Possible Causes
P Wave	
Tall P (P pulmonale)	Right atrial enlargement—dogs
	Left or right atrial enlargement—cats
	Sinus tachycardia—dogs
Wide P (P mitrale)	Left atrial enlargement—dogs and cats
Absent P	"Pseudo" abnormality, look for P waves in other leads
	Hyperkalemia, atrial standstill, silent atrium or atrial fibrillation (look for bumpy baseline)
P height variation	Wandering pacemaker (normal finding particularly with sinus arrhythmia)
	Atrial or junctional premature beats
PR/PQ Interval Duration	
Shortened	High sympathetic tone
	Accessory pathway that by passes the AV node
Prolonged	First-degree AV block
QRS Parameter	
Deep Q wave	Normal variation in deep-chested dogs
	Biventricular enlargement (if other criteria suggestive)
Tall R wave	Left ventricular enlargement
Wide QRS	Ventricular enlargement
	Intraventricular conduction disturbance
Small QRS	Normal variation, pericardial effusion, pleural effusion, pneumothorax, hypothyroidism, obesity
Deep S wave	Normal variation
	Right ventricular enlargement, left ventricular hypertrophy

Continued

Table 3-3.   Summary of Alterations in P-QRS-T Wave Morphology—cont'd

Waveform Alteration	Possible Causes
ST Segment Changes	
Elevation	Myocardial hypoxia, pericardial effusion, pericarditis Digoxin toxicity, transmural myocardial infarction
Depression	Myocardial hypoxia, digoxin toxicity, potassium imbalance Subendocardial myocardial infarction
QT Segment Duration	
Prolongation	Hypokalemia, hypocalcemia, hypothermia, bradycardia Quinidine therapy, conduction disturbance
Shortening	Hyperkalemia, hypercalcemia, digoxin
T Wave	
Large	Myocardial hypoxia, interventricular conduction disturbance, bradycardia, ventricular enlargement, and hyperkalemia
Small	Same as for small QRS, normal for cats

Approach to the Electrocardiogram

1. Obtain standard frontal plane leads (I, II, III, aVR, aVL, aVF) in right lateral recumbency.

2. Determine the heart rate: count the number of QRS complexes in 3 seconds and multiply by 20. 30 big boxes at 50 mm/sec paper speed (15 big boxes at 25mm/sec) = 3 seconds.

3. Determine the rhythm. Scan the strip. Is the rate to fast or slow? Are the R-R intervals regular? Do all the Ps and QRS-Ts look similar? Are the Ps and QRS-Ts related to one another?

4. Estimate the mean electrical axis (MEA) using the QRS complex (Figure 3-4). MEA is the average depolarization direction of the ventricles.

   a. Pick the lead with the greatest QRS deflection. The MEA is directed toward the deflection (positive or negative) pole of this lead.

   b. Identify the isoelectric lead (sum of the positive and negative deflections of the QRS is closest to zero). Determine the lead perpendicular to the isoelectric lead. Determine this leads polarity (positive or negative). The MEA is directed toward the positive or negative pole of this lead.

5. Measure the complexes on lead II at 50 mm/sec paper speed (standard convention[*]).

---

[*]50mm/sec paper speed: 1 small box = 0.02 sec. Standard height calibration: 1 cm (10 small boxes or 2 large boxes) = 1 mV. See the text for interpretation of waveforms.

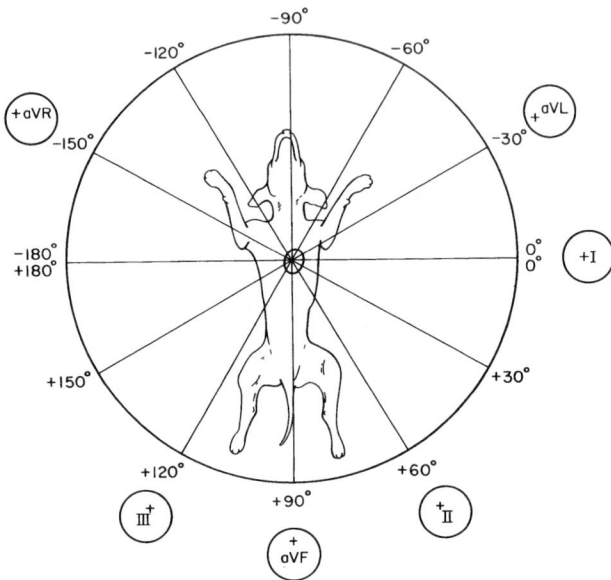

Figure 3-4. The frontal lead system used to estimate MEA. Six leads are shown over a schematic of the ventricles within the thorax of a dog. Each lead is labeled at its positive pole. (*From Tilley LE:* Essentials of Canine and Feline electrocardiography, *ed 3, Philadelphia, 1992, Lea & Febiger.*)

Echocardiography

Echocardiography (heart ultrasound) is used to evaluate the heart and proximal great vessel anatomy noninvasively, and to estimate cardiac function. Three modalities are used in concert to obtain a diagnosis, estimate severity and prognosis, and monitor response to therapy.

Two-Dimensional (Real-Time) Echocardiography

Two-dimensional (2-D) imaging allows visualization of a plane of tissue (depth and width). Imaging is best achieved with perpendicular alignment with tissue interfaces. A variety of standardized imaging planes are obtained from the right and left parasternal locations (Figures 3-5 and 3-6). Anatomic relationships between structures are readily defined. Identification of valvular deformities, masses, pleural and pericardial effusions are more easily appreciated with 2-D imaging. Real-time imaging also facilitates cursor placement for obtaining M-mode and Doppler tracings.

M-Mode Echocardiography

M-mode imaging provides a one-dimensional view (depth) in a localized region of the heart/chambers (Figure 3-7). M-mode displays signals of tissues at known depths (Y axis) across time (X axis). M-mode provides higher resolution of heart walls and chamber interfaces so quantitative measures may be more accurately taken. Many functional indices are acquired with M-mode,

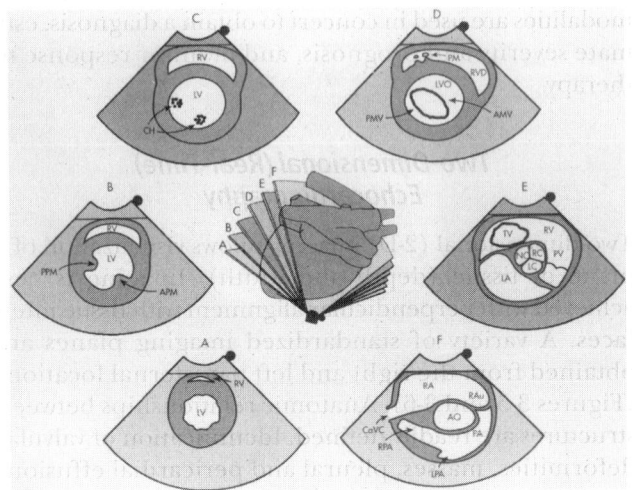

Figure 3-5. Short-axis views obtained from the right parasternal location. (*From Thomas WP et al: J Vet Intern Med 7:247, 1993.*)

such as the percent of fractional shortening, E-point septal separation (estimates of contractility), and aorta–to–left atrial ratio (measure of left atrial size).

Doppler Echocardiography

Doppler echocardiography tracks blood flow through the heart and great vessels. Doppler imaging measures the direction, velocity, and character (laminar versus

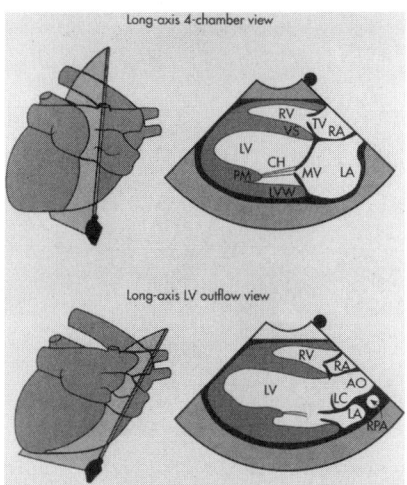

Figure 3-6. Long-axis views obtained from the right parasternal location. (From Thomas WP et al: *J Vet Intem med 7:247, 1993.*)

nonlaminar) of blood flow. Doppler measures can also be converted to pressure using the Bernoulli equation (pressure gradient = $4V^2$, where V = velocity), thus intracardiac pressure measures may be estimated noninvasively. To measure blood flow accurately, parallel cursor alignment with flow must be obtained during Doppler interrogation. Spectral Doppler is displayed as velocity (Y axis) across time (X axis) similar to M-mode display. The direction of blood flow is displayed relative

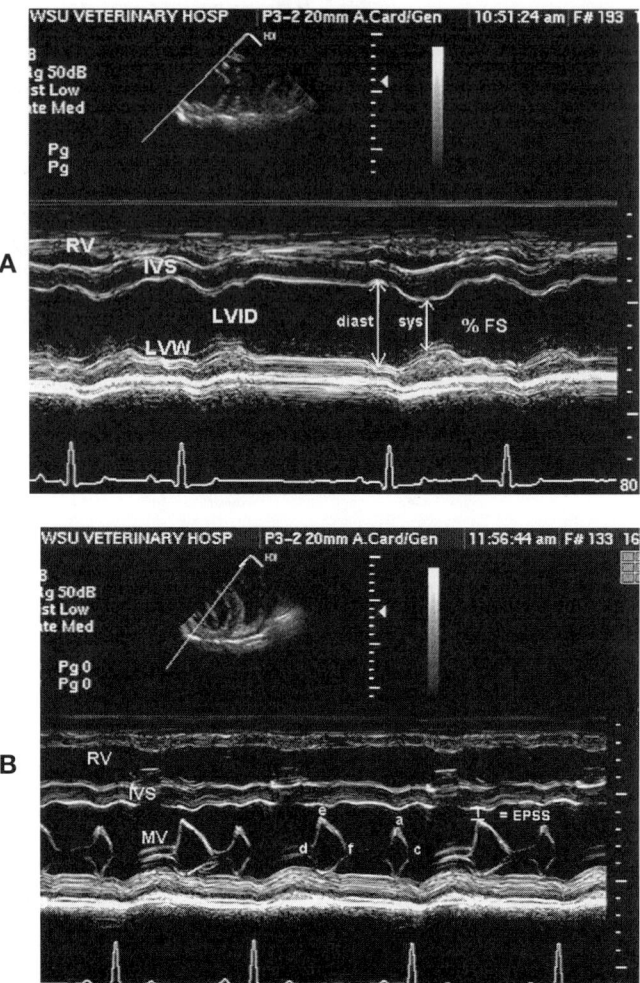

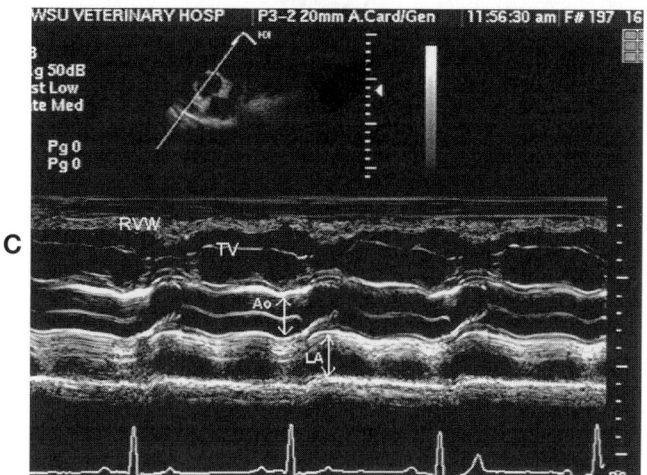

Figure 3-7. Standard M-mode imaging examples. **A,** Note the correct position for cursor placement to obtain measures for percent fractional shortening (%FS) are demonstrated. %FS = LVIDd – LVIDs/ LVIDd × 100. **B,** The anterior mitral valve leaflet looks like the letter M on the M-mode image. The posterior leaflet mirrors the anterior but is more difficult to predictably visualize. The letter designations *D, E, F, A,* and *B* are given to the various points. E-point to septal separation (EPSS) is a common measurement to assess global left ventricular function. **C,** This is an example of appropriate cursor placement for the left atrial *(LA):* aorta *(Ao)* M-mode view. The aortic root is measured at the onset of the QRS, whereas the left atrial measure is taken at the end of systole. LA:Ao ratio of 1-1.2:1 is considered normal. *RVW,* Right ventricular wall; *RV,* right ventricle; *IVS,* interventricular septum; *LVIDd,* left ventricular internal dimension in diastole; *LVIDs,* left ventricular internal dimension in systole; *LVW,* left ventricular wall; *MV,* mitral valve, *TV,* tricuspid valve.

to the transducer (top of the screen). Blood flowing away from the transducer would be recorded below and traveling away from the spectral baseline (Figure 3-8). There are two spectral modalities, pulsed-wave (PW) and continuous-wave (CW) Doppler. PW Doppler uses bursts of ultrasound to interrogate a specific point (designated by the sample volume box). When PW is not sending sound waves, it is receiving the information for display. The biggest disadvantage of PW is that it cannot measure high velocity blood flow. There is a maximum velocity limit (Nyquist limit), after which the velocity display will be ambiguous or aliased. Aliasing does not allow determination of direction or velocity of blood flow (signal recorded above and below the baseline). CW Doppler uses dual crystals so it can transmit and receive simultaneously; therefore, it can measure very high velocity flow. The disadvantage of CW is that it is unable to localize the signal along the beam (no sample box), thus maximal velocities all long the beam are represented. Color flow (CF) Doppler is a form of pulsed-wave Doppler except that it is applied to the anatomic 2-D or M-mode images to assess blood flow. Multiple PW gates are applied to the chosen image, and blood flow is recorded as blue or red (flow away or flow toward the transducer), enhanced or bright blue/red (faster flow), or variance or mixed colors (turbulent flow). Because CF is a form of PW Doppler, it is prone to aliasing, which is displayed as red/blue reversal.

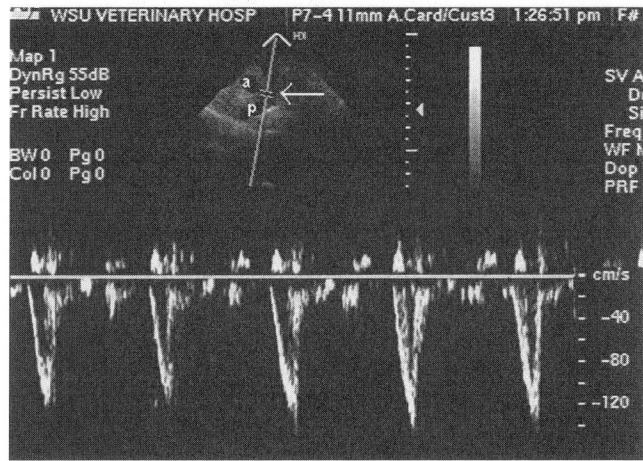

Figure 3-8. Example of normal pulmonic systolic flow in a cat with pulsed-wave Doppler. The sample gate (*arrow*) is at the level of the pulmonic valve. Flow is going away from the transducer into the pulmonary artery *(p)*; thus, the flow is recorded away from the baseline in cm/sec. *a,* Aorta.

Blood Pressure Measurement

Measurement of arterial blood pressure is indicated in patients with renal or endocrine disease, retinal edema or hemorrhages, left ventricular hypertrophy, and systolic myocardial failure and in critically ill patients.

Direct Measurement

Direct arterial pressure measurement is performed by catheterizing an artery and connecting the catheter to a fluid-filled system with a pressure transducer. Although direct arterial pressure measurement is very accurate, it requires more skill to obtain. The procedure is painful for the awake animal, thus sedation or anesthesia is often needed, which may lower the pressure reading.

Indirect Measurement

Noninvasive blood pressure measurement can be accomplished using Doppler or oscillometric techniques. Both techniques use an inflatable cuff placed around a limb or tail to occlude blood flow. Gradual release of cuff pressure is monitored to detect the signal of flow return (systolic pressure value). It is important to choose the appropriate-sized cuff with indirect measurement. The width of the inflatable balloon should be 40% to 50% of the circumference of the limb it is placed. Large cuffs will underestimate and small cuffs will overestimate blood pressure. Typically, a minimum of 5 pressure values are recorded and averaged.

OSCILLOMETRIC METHOD This method uses an automated system for detecting and processing cuff oscillation signals. The cuff is placed around a limb or tail, and the heart rate, systolic, diastolic, and mean blood pressure are automatically recorded. The technique is simple to perform; however, systolic blood pressure may be under-estimated, especially in small dogs and cats, compared with direct measures. Mean pressure values are thought to correlate well with direct measures.

DOPPLER ULTRASONIC METHOD This technique uses the Doppler shift principle to detect blood flow in a superficial artery. The frequency shift is converted to an audible sound (pulsing sound of blood flow). Ultrasonic gel is used to provide good contact between the skin and transducer. The cuff is attached to a pressure manometer and inflated and deflated manually. The first sound heard as the cuff gradually deflates is recorded as the systolic pressure. The diastolic pressure is estimated by a change in the character of the pulsing sound as the cuff deflates. Although the Doppler technique requires slightly more skill and is labor intensive, it is thought to yield accurate systolic pressure results (particularly in small patients).

Normal canine blood pressure: 100/65 to 160/100 (systolic/diastolic)

Normal feline blood pressure: 100/70 to 180/110

Central Venous Pressure Measurement

Central venous pressure (CVP) is an estimate of right atrial pressure. CVP is obtained by aseptically placing a catheter into the jugular vein extending to (or close to) the right atrium. A water manometer (or pressure transducer) is attached to the catheter with extension tubing. The fluid column in the manometer is allowed to equilibrate with the patient's CVP. Normal CVP in dogs and cats is 0 to 10 cm H_2O (or 0 to 8 mm Hg). CVP measurement is useful in identifying elevated right heart filling pressures or to monitor patients receiving large volumes of fluid.

Holter Monitor (Continuous Ambulatory Electrocardiography)

Holter monitor recording is indicated in patients with intermittent weakness or collapse in which an arrhythmia is suspected. Holter monitoring is sometimes used to pre-screen certain breeds for arrhythmic forms of cardiomyopathy (Boxers and Dobermans). The recorder is lightweight and can be easily worn by most patients as a "backpack." The ECG is recorded on a cassette tape or digital flash card. Experienced personnel and computer analysis systems programmed for veterinary patients is crucial to accurate data. Alternatively, the full disclosed report may be manually analyzed by experienced persons.

Cardiac Catheterization

Cardiac catheterization involves placement of specialized catheters into the heart and great vessels for pressure measurement, angiography, obtaining blood gas samples, measuring cardiac output, and performing interventions. General anesthesia is typically required. Many disorders that once required catheterization for diagnosis may now be reliably evaluated with noninvasive echocardiography. Today, cardiac catheterization is primarily reserved for those patients requiring interventional procedures, such as balloon valvuloplasty, pacemaker implantation, or coil embolization of an unwanted vessel.

Special Tests

Computed tomography (CT) and magnetic resonance imaging (MRI) are noninvasive techniques that may provide additional information regarding cardiovascular disorders. In some cases, detection of thrombi, masses (particularly of the heart base), pericardial disorders, and certain complex congenital anomalies may be better defined with MRI or CT. MRI usually provides better tissue characterization than CT and may be used to assess blood flow. Because of the cost and need for general anesthesia, these tests are not often first-line diagnostic techniques.

4

Principles of Therapy for Congestive Heart Failure

Pathophysiology Overview

When the heart cannot adequately meet the demands of the body for oxygen and nutrients, the heart is said to be "failing." Heart failure is a syndrome manifest by many different cardiac pathologies; thus heart failure alone does not imply a specific etiology. Abnormal myocardial contractility may be an underlying cause of heart failure (i.e., dilated cardiomyopathy), but it can also be a consequence of another process (chronic volume overload i.e., mitral regurgitation). Heart failure can also occur when the myocardial contractility is normal. As the cardiac abnormality progresses, the body activates several compensatory mechanisms to attempt to maintain adequate forward blood flow. These mechanisms may support the circulation initially but chronically lead to the clinical signs of heart failure and accelerate progression of cardiac disease. When these mechanisms cause fluid accumulation (pulmonary edema, pleural effusion, or ascites), *clinical congestive heart failure* (CHF) is present.

Understanding the basic pathophysiologic causes of heart disease is essential to understanding the strategies for therapy. Although some disorders may have features of more than one group (especially chronic conditions), they are typically classified according to the primary underlying abnormality (Table 4-1).

Compensatory Mechanisms

As cardiac output declines, compensatory mechanisms are activated to increase the heart rate and peripheral vascular resistance, and retain fluid volume. These mechanisms enhance cardiac output and maintain arterial blood pressure. As stated earlier, these changes may be helpful in the initial stages of cardiac disease but become detrimental to the heart over time. Many medical therapies are designed to antagonize these mechanisms. Common neurohormonal changes include increases in sympathetic nervous tone, activation of the renin-angiotension-aldosterone system (RAAS), and release of antidiuretic hormone (vasopressin). Some endogenous mechanisms such as atrial natriuretic peptide (ANP) oppose the bad effects of RAAS. ANP enhances natriuresis (and reduces fluid volume) in response to stretch of the atria. Figure 4-1 summarizes the neurohormonal compensatory mechanisms and their effects in heart failure.

Treatment of Congestive Heart Failure

Many therapeutic goals are common to all underlying causes of heart failure. In general, it is desirable to improve cardiac output, control edema or effusions, reduce the cardiac workload, control arrhythmias, and avoid complications such as renal compromise. The strategies chosen to achieve these goals are commonly dependent on the underlying pathophysiologic heart failure group and the severity of the individual's disease. Table 4-2 summarizes practical therapy for cardiac patients based on known cardiac pathology.

Diuretics

Diuretics are commonly a *first-line therapy* in the management of CHF. Diuretics aide in removing excess fluid

Table 4-1. Pathophysiologic Groups of Heart Disease

Classification	Pathophysiology	Example
Myocardial failure	Diseases that result in heart muscle weakness are included here. Contractility (systolic function) is generally poor; valvular insufficiency may be a secondary finding.	Dilated cardiomyopathy (classic example) Chronic volume overloading diseases (see below) Myocarditis (viral, bacterial, immune-mediated, toxic)
Volume overload	Diseases of volume overload to the heart cause chamber dilation (eccentric hypertrophy) of the affected region or regions but usually exhibit normal systolic function. In some cases, contractility may decline with time and progressive increases in heart wall stress occur. "Cardiomyopathy of overload" is sometimes used to describe this phenomenon.	Valvular insufficiency (mitral, tricuspid, aortic insufficiency) AV shunts (patent ductus arteriosis, ventricular septal defect) Chronic anemia (fluid-retaining process)
Pressure overload	Diseases that impair or obstruct ventricular ejection cause an excessive pressure generation by the ventricle. Pressure overloads stimulate concentric myocardial hypertrophy. The hypertrophied myocardium is stiffer than normal and relaxes (diastolic function) poorly. The thickened heart walls may outstrip their blood supply, and myocardial ischemia and ventricular arrhythmias may result.	Subaortic stenosis Pulmonic stenosis Systemic hypertension Pulmonary hypertension

| Diastolic dysfunction | Diseases that oppose ventricular filling also result in abnormal diastolic function. Although this category has some features in common with pressure overload diseases, reduced ventricular compliance is a primary abnormality and not secondary to pressure overload. | Hypertrophic cardiomyopathy Restrictive cardiomyopathy Pericardial effusion Constrictive pericardial disease |
| Arrhythmias | Persistent tachyarrhythmias or bradyarrhythmias can also lead to heart failure. Myocardial ischemia and fluid volume retention are common findings. | Supraventricular tachycardia (e.g., atrial fibrillation, atrial tachycardia) Ventricular tachycardia Bradyarrhythmias (e.g., second-degree and third-degree heart block, sick sinus syndrome) |

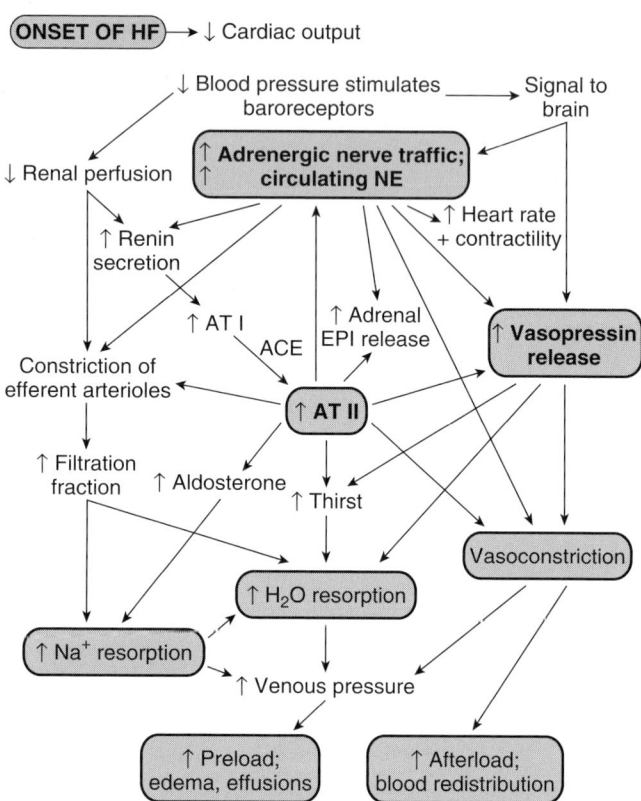

Figure 4-1. Summary of the neurohormonal compensatory mechanisms and their effects in heart failure. ATI, Agniotenisin I; AT II, angiotensin II. (*From Ware WA: Aproximate locations, murmur shapes, neurohormonal mechanisms. In Nelson RW, Couto CG, eds: Small animal internal medicine, ed 2, St. Louis, 1998, Mosby.*)

from lungs and the vascular system, thus decreasing congestion and edema. Loop diuretics (e.g., furosemide, bumetanide) working directly on the nephron loop of Henle are primarily used because of their potency. Other diuretics are sometimes combined with furosemide in the chronic CHF patient such as spironolactone (a potassium-sparing diuretic) and hydrochlorothiazide (a thiazide diuretic). These diuretics are weaker than loop diuretics but may have an additive effect in refractory cases of pulmonary edema or pleural effusion.

Vasodilators

Vasodilators can improve cardiac output and reduce fluid accumulations in CHF patients. *Venodilators* relax systemic veins, which increases their capacitance and reduces cardiac preload or filling pressure. This strategy (i.e., cutaneous nitroglycerin, isosorbide dinitrate) is often used in acute or severe left-sided CHF to shift more blood into the venous system and reduce pulmonary congestion. *Arteriolar dilators* relax arteriolar smooth muscle, thus decreasing systemic vascular resistance (and blood pressure), and reducing afterload (enhancing forward output). Arterial dilation (using amlodipine, hydralazine, nitroprusside) is often sought in cases of acute or severe mitral regurgitation and CHF to enhance forward movement of blood and decrease backward movement (mitral regurgitation). *Mixed*

Table 4-2. Practical Cardiac Therapy for Patients Based on Pathophysiology

Heart Disease Group	Goal	Suggested Therapy
Myocardial failure (systolic failure)	1. Improve cardiac output (+ inotropes, vasodilators) 2. ↓ edema and effusions (diuretics, vasodilators, diet) 3. Reduce cardiac workload (rest, vasodilators) 4. Avoid renal compromise 5. Control arrhythmias, if present (e.g., in Dobermans, Boxers)	1. Digoxin, dopamine, dobutamine 2 and 3. Lasix, spironolactone, hydrochlorothiazide, ACEi (e.g., enalapril, benazepril, lisinopril) 4. Monitor laboratory work, blood pressure 5. Administer lidocaine, procainamide, mexiletine, sotalol, and others

Diastolic failure (restricted filling) pericardial disease, HCM, RCM*	1. Drain pericardial fluid, remove pericardium if need, treat underlying disease
	2. a. ↑ Cardiac filling, slow heart rate
	  b. Enhance myocardial perfusion and slow heart rate
	  c. ↓ Edema and effusions
	  d. Control arrhythmias
	  e. Avoid embolic complications
		1. Pericardiocentesis, etc.
		2. a. Beta blockers, calcium channel blockers
		  b. i.e., Atenolol, diltiazem
		  c. Lasix, spironolactone, diet
		  d. Procainamide, beta blockers (cats)
		  e. Aspirin, heparins

Volume overload	1. ↓ Edema and effusion 2. ↓ Valve regurgitation 3. Decrease cardiac workload (rest, vasodilators) 4. Improve forward output (vasodilators) 5. If systolic cysfunction occurs, administer positive inotropes	1. Diuretics, ACEi, diet 2. ACEi, amlodipine, hydralazine 3 and 4. ACEi, amlodipine, hydralazine, and rest 5. Digoxin, dopamine, dobutamine

Pressure overload	1. Relieve stenosis, if possible	1. Valvuloplasty
	2. Reduce arteriolar hypertension	2. Amlodipine, atenolol, ACEi
	3. Enhance myocardial filling, perfusion and slow heart rate (through beta blockers, calcium channel blockers)	3. Diltiazem, atenolol
	4. Control edema, effusions, arrhythmias	4. Diuretics, ACEi Antiarrhythmics: lidocaine, sotalol, procainamide, mexiletine, tocainide, others

ACEi, Angiotensin-converting enzyme inhibitors; RCM, restrictive cardiomyopathy; HCM, hypertrophilcardiomyopathy.
*Some RCM behave as systolic dysfunction.

vasodilators are associated with both venous and arteriolar dilation. Of this category, *angiotensin-converting enzyme inhibitors (ACEis)* are used almost exclusively. In addition to their vasodilation effect, they reduce sodium and water retention through their ability to decrease aldosterone secretion. Indirectly, ACEis decrease adrenergic nervous system tone and have been shown to retard myocardial fibrosis. Because of their multiple beneficial effects, ACEis are considered the vasodilator of choice in most heart failure patients. Popular preparations include enalapril, benazepril, and lisinopril. Systemic blood pressures must be carefully monitored with vasodilation (especially arteriodilation).

Positive Inotropes

Drugs that *improve the force of contraction* are indicated particularly when systolic dysfunction is documented. These drugs increase intracellular calcium in the myocyte through different mechanisms. The increased calcium available to the contractile proteins is responsible for the inotropic effect. The oral preparation of digoxin is the most routinely used positive inotrope in patients with CHF. Digoxin is also thought to improve baroreceptor function and alterations in sympathetic nervous system tone in CHF patients. Another clinical use of digoxin is as an antiarrhythmic agent for supraventricular arrhythmias (to slow atrioventricular

[AV] node conduction), especially atrial fibrillation. The catecholamines, dopamine and dobutamine (synthetic form), act by binding to cardiac beta$_1$ adrenergic receptors to cause an increase in cytosolic calcium. These therapies are given by continuous rate infusion and are usually reserved for the patient with acute or severe CHF presentation with systolic dysfunction. Dopamine in low doses stimulates splanchnic dopamine receptors and can also be used to enhance renal perfusion through this mechanism. Amrinone and milrinone are phosphodiesterase inhibitors, which act indirectly to increase intracellular calcium. They are rarely used in veterinary patients.

Negative Inotropes

Negative inotropic or chronotropic therapies are indicated in some patients in whom diastolic dysfunction is the underlying cause of the CHF. Impaired filling during diastole leads to a reduced ejection during systole. A classic example is feline hypertrophic cardiomyopathy (HCM). Tachyarrhythmias (i.e., atrial fibrillation) may also impair diastolic filling, either alone or in conjunction with other disease processes. In certain situations, a beta blocker (e.g., atenolol) or a calcium channel blocker (e.g., diltiazem) may be used to slow down the heart rate, increase diastolic filling time, promote myocardial perfusion, and thus enhance forward output.

Diets and Supplements

Heart failure patients have tendency to retain sodium and fluid (neurohumoral effects). Therefore diets low in sodium are generally recommended. In many patients with mild or early heart disease, moderate sodium restriction is adequate. This can be accomplished by the use of some senior-type diets and avoiding high-salt treats. As disease progresses, increasing sodium restriction with diets such as Hills KD or Purina NF is advised. In severe refractory cases of heart failure, Hills HD and Purina CV (more sodium restriction) may be used. It is important that the patient maintain adequate caloric intake. Feeding nutritionally balanced, highly bioavailable foods may help combat the effects of cardiac cachexia seen in some chronic CHF patients.

Supplements such as carnitine, taurine, coenzyme Q (and others) have not been extensively studied in clinical trials. However, there does appear to be a beneficial effect in administering taurine and carnitine in some breeds of dogs with dilated cardiomyopathy. American Cocker Spaniels, some golden retrievers, and some lines of Boxer dogs may partially regress their myocardial changes with carnitine and taurine supplementation. A plasma taurine level can be analyzed, and administration of both dietary additives can be attempted. Altered amino acid composition is suspected to be a consequence (as opposed to a cause) of the myocardial disease in dogs. It is not known why some dogs benefit from supplementation.

Emergency Management of Congestive Heart Failure

Patients that present with severe respiratory distress from fulminant CHF (pulmonary edema +/– pleural and abdominal effusions) are not candidates for multiple immediate tests and manipulations. These animals are severely stressed. Unnecessary handling should be avoided until the patient is sufficiently stable for additional diagnostics or techniques. The test of greatest value in the respiratory patient is thoracic radiography. Radiography quickly localizes the problem to cardiac, airway, pulmonary parenchyma, or pleural space disease. This test further narrows the differential diagnosis and aides to establish a diagnostic plan. Figure 4-2 describes strategies that may be used in initial management of the severe CHF patient.

Monitoring the Patient with Congestive Heart Failure

The key to successful management of the CHF patient is frequent monitoring and adjustment of treatment strategies. Serially evaluating respiratory rate and effort,

Record: character of respiration (inspiratory, expiratory effort), respiratory rate, mucous membrane color, CRT, abdominal effusions, peripheral pulses, jugular veins, heart rate and rhythm, heart and lung sounds, etc.

Assess the patient's ability to withstand handling for a diagnostic test.

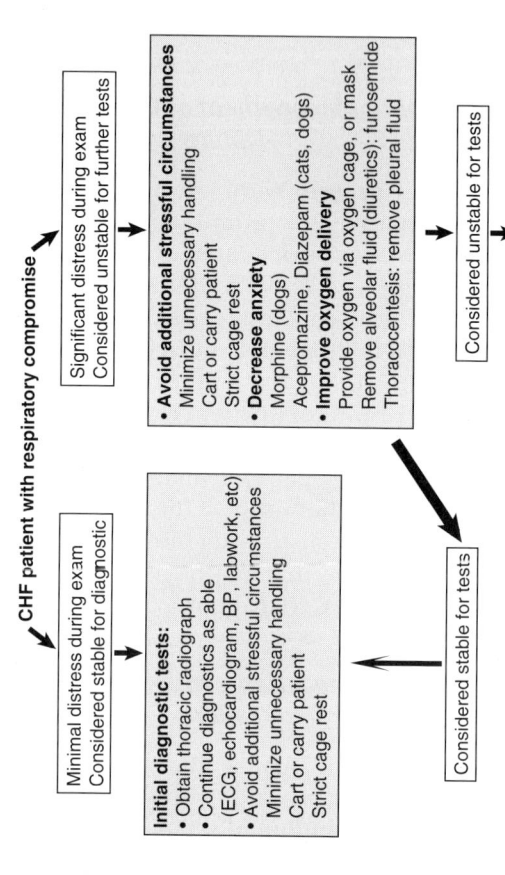

CHF patient with respiratory compromise

Minimal distress during exam
Considered stable for diagnostic

Significant distress during exam
Considered unstable for further tests

Initial diagnostic tests:
• Obtain thoracic radiograph
• Continue diagnostics as able (ECG, echocardiogram, BP, labwork, etc)
• Avoid additional stressful circumstances
Minimize unnecessary handling
Cart or carry patient
Strict cage rest

• **Avoid additional stressful circumstances**
Minimize unnecessary handling
Cart or carry patient
Strict cage rest
• **Decrease anxiety**
Morphine (dogs)
Acepromazine, Diazepam (cats, dogs)
• **Improve oxygen delivery**
Provide oxygen via oxygen cage, or mask
Remove alveolar fluid (diuretics): furosemide
Thoracocentesis: remove pleural fluid

Considered unstable for tests

Considered stable for tests

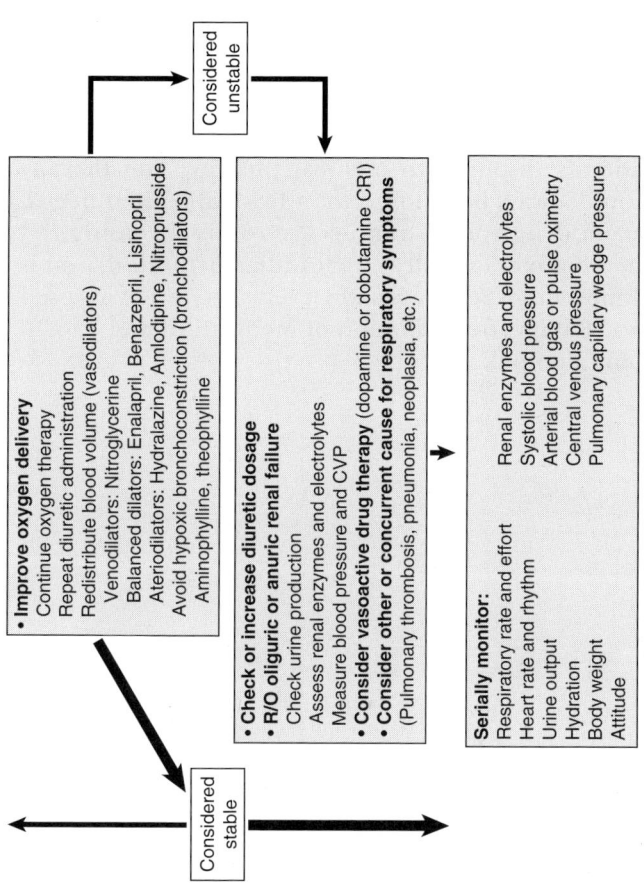

Figure 4-2. Algorithm used in the initial management of severe or acute CHF.

heart rate and rhythm, kidney function and electrolytes, and blood pressure are recommended as minimal monitoring parameters. Recheck examinations may be scheduled every few days initially, to every few months, depending on the severity of the disease and the patient's response to medical therapy. The therapy should always be tailored to individual patient needs. Serum drug concentrations are routinely monitored when digoxin (as well as some antiarrhythmic drugs) is administered. Serum digoxin levels are typically assessed 7 to 10 days after initiation of medication and 8 to 10 hours after pill.

5

Canine Myocardial Diseases

Dilated Cardiomyopathy

Definition

Dilated cardiomyopathy (DCM) is characterized by poor myocardial contractility and cardiac chamber enlargement. The disease is often progressive, and patients may present with congestive heart failure (CHF).

Cause

DCM is often considered a primary heart disease of unknown etiology. Genetic factors are implicated because DCM is prevalent in certain breeds and breed lines of dogs. Common breeds in which DCM is found are Doberman Pinschers, Boxers, American Cocker Spaniels, Great Danes, Newfoundlands, golden retrievers, Wolfhounds, and other large or giant breeds of dogs. Potential causes of secondary dilated cardiomyopathy are toxins (doxorubicin, ethyl alcohol), malnutrition, myocarditis or severe systemic inflammatory disease (granulomatous, neoplastic, sepsis), and possibly endocrinopathies (hypothyroidism, diabetes mellitus). With the exception of toxin-induced DCM, many secondary causes of DCM do not present with clinical CHF.

Pathophysiology

Poor myocardial contractility (systolic dysfunction) is the functional defect in this disease. Cardiac chamber enlargement or dilation occurs secondary to the impaired pump function and output. Progressive chamber enlargements and muscle dysfunction often lead to atrioventricular (AV) valve insufficiency, which may accelerate cardiac chamber dilation. Increased diastolic stiffness of the diseased muscle also contributes to elevated end-diastolic pressures. Increased filling pressures and venous congestion ultimately lead to congestive heart failure. Compensatory mechanisms were discussed earlier.

Clinical Presentation

Lethargy, weakness, and exercise intolerance (signs of poor forward output) are common earlier in the disease state. However, these signs may be dismissed in sedentary, older patients. Tachypnea, dyspnea and coughing (if left-sided CHF), or abdominal distension or ascites (if right-sided CHF) are typical presenting complaints. Some dogs present with the history of intermittent collapse or syncope due to ventricular arrhythmias (especially Boxers). Physical examination findings depend on the degree of heart failure. Tachycardia, pale mucous membranes, and delayed capillary refill time (CRT) (peripheral vasoconstriction) are the result of increased sympathetic tone seen in heart failure. Jugular venous distension and pulsations indicate elevated right heart filling pressures. Peripheral pulses may be weak, variable in strength, or demonstrate deficits if arrhythmias are present. The heart rhythm may also be irregular if ventricular arrhythmias or atrial fibrillation are present. Heart sounds can be muffled secondary to pleural effusion. Soft mitral or tricuspid murmurs are sometimes noted but are not consistent findings. The S_3 gallop sound (rapid filling vibration of a dilated ventricle) is classic for DCM, but again is inconsistent. Pulmonary crackles may be heard with left-sided CHF, or sometimes the lung sounds seem especially harsh or loud, or quieter than normal. Not all dogs with DCM demonstrate clinical signs. Owing to noninvasive echocardiography, increasing numbers of occult and asymptomatic DCM cases are diagnosed.

Diagnosis

Thoracic radiographs may reveal generalized cardiomegaly (classic), but some dogs have only minimal enlargement or primarily left atrial enlargement (especially Doberman Pinschers). Pulmonary interstitial opacities, particularly in the hilar and caudodorsal regions, and engorged pulmonary veins are often noted if left-sided CHF has occurred. Pleural effusion, enlarged caudal vena cava, hepatosplenomegaly, and ascites are common sequelae of right-sided CHF.

Electrocardiographic findings can be variable. The electrocardiogram (ECG) may appear normal or demonstrate a widened QRS complex with a sloppy R descent (classic). A prolonged P wave (P mitrale) typically indicates left atrial enlargement. Other left ventricular enlargement patterns or QRS conduction abnormalities may be found. Ventricular premature beats or paroxysmal ventricular tachycardia may be found in many patients with DCM but is especially prominent in Boxers and Doberman Pinschers. Atrial fibrillation is also commonly noted, particularly in giant breeds, such as wolfhounds.

Echocardiography is the most sensitive, noninvasive test to assess cardiac chamber sizes and estimate systolic and diastolic function. Dilation of all four chambers is classic, with the left-sided chambers predominating. Ventricular wall thickness is normal to decreased. Occasionally, minimal chamber dilation is present, but poor systolic or diastolic function is noted (e.g., percentage of fractional shortening, ejection fraction, mitral valve E-point septal separation [EPSS], the ratio of the mitral valve Doppler signal E wave to the A wave [E/A ratio] reversal of the mitral valve Doppler envelope) (Figure 5-1).

Therapy

Therapy is aimed at eliminating the signs of congestive failure, increasing cardiac output (see Chapter 4) and controlling arrhythmias. Oral positive inotropic support with digoxin is most commonly used, however, in a critical setting, Dopamine or dobutamine may be used as a continuous rate infusion. Digoxin is also used to slow the ventricular response rate to atrial fibrillation.

Loop diuretics and angiotensin-converting enzyme inhibitors (ACEis) are administered to combat congestion, effusions or edema, and improve forward output. ACEis may also have additional effects such as retarding myocardial remodeling and fibrosis. Antiarrhythmics are used when moderate to severe ventricular arrhythmias are present, as well as in breeds known to be at risk for sudden death (Boxers, Dobermans). L-Carnitine and taurine supplementation have shown some beneficial

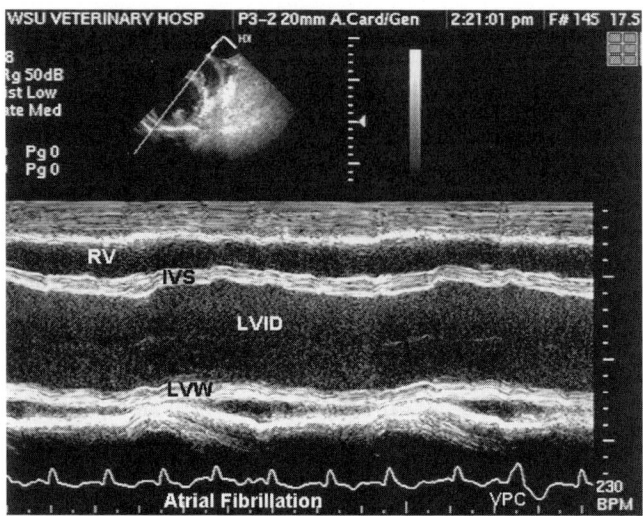

Figure 5-1. A left ventricular M-mode image obtained from a Springer Spaniel with DCM. Note dilation of the ventricular chamber and poor motion of the IVS and LV wall during systole (compare with Fig. 3-7, *A*). This patient's heart rhythm is atrial fibrillation.

effects in American Cocker Spaniels and some retrievers. A whole blood taurine level may be assessed, and administration of both supplements may be tried. Many Cocker Spaniels show improvement in their myocardial function tests within 3 to 6 months.

Patient Monitoring

The aggressiveness of therapy and monitoring depends on the severity of heart failure and other complications such as kidney failure. Renal enzymes, electrolytes, systolic blood pressure, serum digoxin levels, ECG, and antiarrhythmic drug levels are common parameters to evaluate. Reexamination may be suggested every 1 to 3 weeks initially, then every 2 to 6 months, depending on the individual.

Specific Breed Considerations

Boxers have a form of DCM that is primarily characterized by arrhythmias and sudden death. These dogs may have no clinical, radiographic, or echocardiographic signs of heart disease. The arrhythmias may be picked up on a physical examination, or owners might complain of sudden weakness or collapse in their pet. At present, Holter monitoring is the best means to evaluate the dogs. Because of the uniqueness of DCM in this breed, it is commonly referred to as *Boxer dysrhythmia syndrome* or *Boxer cardiomyopathy.*

Dobermans may also have severe ventricular arrhythmias and sudden death. However, left-sided CHF is equally as common. Milder radiographic cardiomegaly (compared with other large and giant breeds) is often present, with some patients demonstrating only mild left atrial enlargement.

American Cocker Spaniels and some retrievers may respond to supplementation with taurine and L-carnitine (see previous section).

Hypertrophic Cardiomyopathy

Primary hypertrophic cardiomyopathy (HCM) is rare in dogs (in contrast to cats). Left ventricular hypertrophy in dogs is usually the result of a pressure-overload state (i.e., subaortic stenosis or systemic hypertension). In HCM, left ventricular hypertrophy causes the chamber to become stiff and noncompliant. Systolic function is normal but relaxation and filling (diastolic function) is impaired. HCM is diagnosed occasionally in male, large breed sporting dogs. Diagnosis and treatment are similar to that for feline HCM.

Myocarditis

Injury to the myocardium can occur as a result of trauma, invasion of infectious organisms, toxins or inflammatory mediators or by the patient's immune response (Box 5-1). Presentation is usually related to underlying disease process versus cardiac disease, although fatal ventricular arrhythmias are not uncommon. Cardiac diagnostic tests may appear similar to DCM. Therapy is aimed at the underlying cause, and severe arrhythmias are treated with antiarrhythmic drugs.

Box 5-1. Proposed Causes of Myocarditis

Trauma or contusions
Viral: parvovirus, others?
Bacterial: many organisms
Lyme disease: *Borrelia burgdorferi* (regional)
Protozoal: *Trypanosoma cruzi, Toxoplasma gondii, Neosporum caninum, Hepatozoon canis*
Fungal: *Cryptococcus, Coccidiodes, Histoplasma, Aspergillus, Blastomycoses*
Rickettsial: *Rickettsia rickettsii, Ehrlichia canis, Bartonella elizabethae*

Traumatic Myocarditis

Blunt trauma to the thorax may result in cardiac (usually ventricular) arrhythmias. These rhythms may be caused by alterations in nervous system tone, ischemia and reperfusion, or electrolyte and acid-base disturbances. The rhythm disturbances are often noted 24 to 72 hours after insult. Indications for treatment of ventricular arrhythmias are given in Box 5-2.

Box 5-2.   Indications for Treatment of Ventricular Rhythms

Frequent ventricular premature contractions (VPCs) of more than 20 to 30 per minute

VPCs in pairs or paroxysms at a rate greater than 120 per minute

Multiform VPCs

R on T phenomenon

Clinical signs of low output

Known myocardial failure

High-risk breed for sudden death (Boxers, Dobermans)

6

Feline Myocardial Diseases

Hypertrophic cardiomyopathy (HCM) is the most common acquired heart disease in the feline patient. Recent information suggests that HCM is inherited as a dominant trait in certain breeds of cats. In addition to HCM, other myocardial diseases may be identified in the cat. It is important to understand the underlying disease process in the feline patient, because treatments for the different cardiomyopathies vary with the type (i.e., HCM therapy differs from dilated cardiomyopathy [DCM]).

Hypertrophic Cardiomyopathy

Definition and Cause (Primary Disease)

Idiopathic left ventricular hypertrophy is documented through echocardiography. Genetic mutations of contractile proteins, increased myocardial sensitivity to catecholamines, and collagen, calcium, or other hormonal abnormalities have all been postulated etiologies. There appears to be a familial incidence in the Maine Coon and possibly the Persian cat. Others breeds reported to be at increased risk are American and British Shorthair cats; however, the disease is frequently noted to occur in common domestic short and longhair cats. The incidence of HCM is greater in middle-aged male cats.

Definition and Cause (Secondary Disease)

Left ventricular hypertrophy may result from increases in afterload, chronic high output states, and hormones acting as growth factors. When underlying causes are responsible for the ventricular hypertrophy, *secondary HCM* is said to be present. Hyperthyroidism, systemic hypertension (i.e., chronic renal failure), hypersomatotropism, and occasional infiltrative diseases (lymphoma) are reported causes of secondary HCM.

Pathophysiology

Hypertrophy causes increased ventricular stiffness, poor compliance, and poor relaxation (diastolic dysfunction) of the heart muscle. Because ventricular hypertrophy may outstrip the available myocardial blood supply, ischemia, and fibrosis of the subendocardial regions further exacerbate chamber stiffness characteristics. Hypertrophy of the interventricular septum may create left ventricular outflow obstruction and worsen the hypertrophic response, as well as severely limit cardiac output. When outflow obstruction is present, the disease may be recharacterized as *hypertrophic obstructive cardiomyopathy (HOCM)*. Left atrial enlargement develops as the atrium encounters high diastolic filling pressures when it contracts against the stiff, noncompliant left ventricle. When left atrial (and pulmonary venous) pressures cause excessive pulmonary capillary hydrostatic pressure and pulmonary parenchymal fluid exudation, left-sided heart failure (pulmonary edema) occurs.

Clinical Presentation

Most pets present with respiratory symptoms because exercise intolerance is difficult to assess in cats. Tachypnea, dyspnea, and panting are typical if pulmonary edema or pleural effusion are present. In contrast to dogs, cats may develop pleural effusion with left heart failure as well as right heart failure. Cough is an uncommon symptom in cats with congestive heart failure (CHF). Coughing cats should be evaluated for airway disease. Patients may present with paralysis or paresis of a single limb or both rear limbs if arterial thrombus has occurred. The temperature of the affected limb or limbs should be compared with the normal limbs by palpation. Likewise, the arterial pulses of the hindlimbs (or forelimbs) should be evaluated simultaneously for strength and character. Syncope is occasionally reported as a first symptom (presumed arrhythmias).

PHYSICAL EXAMINATION   Auscultation usually reveals a systolic ejection murmur over the left ventricular outflow tract area (left sternal, heart base). Mitral regurgitation may be ausculted at the left apex. A gallop sound resulting from atrial contraction may be heard best on the left (S_4 gallop). Even with significant pulmonary edema, cats often have quiet lung sounds. Auscultation can underestimate the severity of heart failure in the feline species. Attention to respiratory rate and character of respirations may yield more helpful information. Muffled heart and lung sounds ventrally can indicate pleural effusion. Jugular pulses may be noted when right heart filling pressures are elevated. Weak or absent femoral pulses may be documented with severely compromised cardiac output.

Diagnostics

THORACIC RADIOGRAPHS The cardiac silhouette may be normal in some cases of HCM or appear small. Concentric hypertrophy is not as consistently identified as cardiomegaly on the chest radiograph (as is eccentric hypertrophy). Left atrial +/− left ventricular enlargement may be noted in many cases. Pulmonary vascular engorgement (especially veins) may be found in patients with CHF or "pre-failure." Patchy diffuse or focal interstitial patterns are common if left-sided CHF has developed. Pleural effusion in the cat may represent left or biventricular failure.

ELECTROCARDIOGRAPHY The electrocardiogram (ECG) may be normal, or left ventricular enlargement patterns may be present. Supraventricular and especially ventricular arrhythmias are not uncommon. Occasionally, high-grade second-degree heart block or complete heart block may be responsible for syncope.

ECHOCARDIOGRAPHY Echocardiography is the best means of diagnosis and determination of severity of hypertrophy (Figure 6-1). Concentric hypertrophy is usual. However, some cats demonstrate only hypertrophy of the interventricular septum (asymmetric septal hypertrophy [ASH]) +/− papillary muscles. Outflow obstruction caused by the hypertrophied septum and papillary muscles may be identified by systolic anterior motion of the mitral valve (SAM) on the M-mode

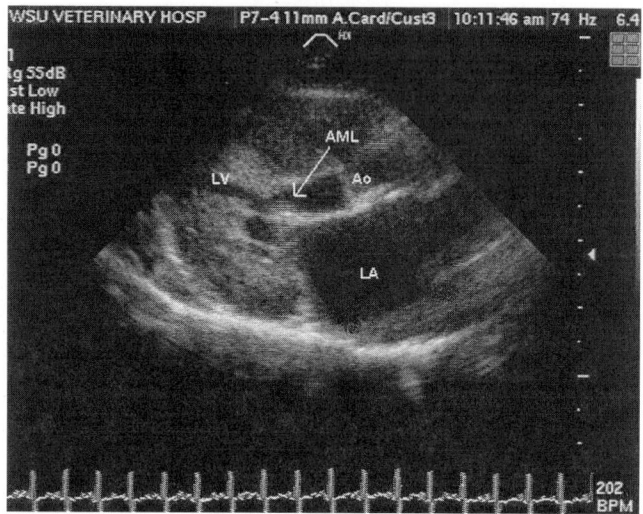

Figure 6-1. This echocardiogram image was obtained from a 7-year-old male, domestic long-hair cat with hypertrophic obstructive cardiomyopathy (HOCM). Note the prominent left ventricular hypertrophy, left atrial dilation, and thickening of the anterior mitral valve (AML) leaflet due to the trauma from the forces pulling the valve toward the septum in systole.

examination (Figure 6-2). In this scenario, the mitral valve is pulled into the outflow tract during systole, and mitral regurgitation may be noted. Left atrial enlargement (LAE) is typical, and thrombi may be found within the body of the left atrium or auricle.

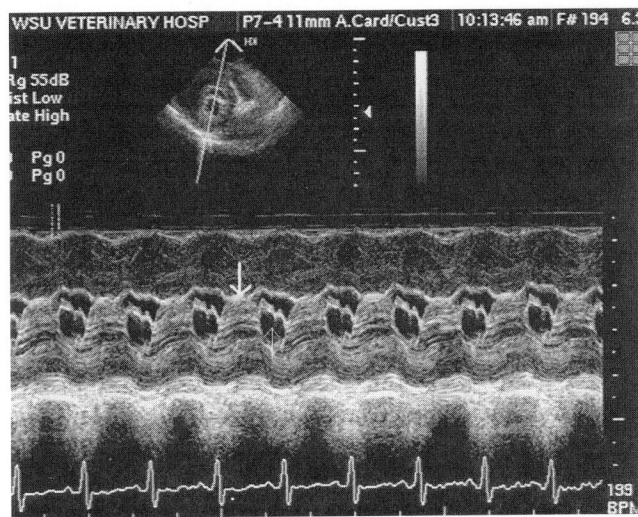

Figure 6-2. This is a M-mode image taken at the level of the mitral valve from the same cat as in Figure 6-1. The mitral valve is indicated with the thin arrow. The thick arrow demonstrates the systolic anterior movement (SAM) of the mitral valve as it is pulled into the outflow tract due to the suction created with septal hypertrophy in HOCM.

Therapeutic Goals for Hypertrophic Cardiomyopathy

Positive inotropes (digoxin) and arterial dilation (hydralazine, amlodipine) are *contraindicated,* particularly if outflow obstruction is suspected (Table 6-1). ACE

Table 6.1. Therapeutic Goals for Hypertrophic Cardiomyopathy

Goals	Drug Therapy
Slow heart rate	Beta blockers or calcium channel blockers (Atenolol, Diltiazem)
Improve ventricular filling and relaxation	
Enhance myocardial perfusion (longer diastole)	
Decrease myocardial workload	
Promote excretion of sodium and fluid in CHF	Furosemide
	Enalapril (particularly if right-sided CHF)
	Spironolactone +/− hydrochlorothiazide in refractory CHF cases
Avoid thromboembolism	Aspirin, warfarin?
	Low-molecular-weight heparins (under investigation)

inhibitors are controversial for routine administration. However, patients with refractory pleural effusions may benefit. In *secondary HCM,* treatment for the underlying condition may be the only necessary intervention.

Patient Monitoring

Renal enzymes, electrolytes, blood pressure, ECG, and left ventricular hypertrophy changes are common parameters to evaluate. Reexamination may be suggested every 1 to 3 weeks initially, depending on severity of disease, then every 3 to 6 months. The *prognosis* is variable and often depends on the response to therapy as well as concurrent problems (i.e., renal disease). Many cats will maintain a good quality of life for several years after diagnosis.

Special Considerations

Many cats present with "occult" disease. Murmurs may be found incidentally on routine exams performed for another purpose. The decision to intervene prophylactically may be based on the finding of LAE, left ventricular wall thickness greater than 6 mm, left ventricular outflow obstruction, or significant arrhythmias. At a minimum, reexaminations are suggested to assess progression of hypertrophy, but progression is not necessarily inevitable.

Restrictive Cardiomyopathy

Cause and Pathophysiology

RCM is characterized by extensive myocardial (especially subendocardial) fibrosis. The etiology is not known, but many underlying pathologies may lead to this abnormality (e.g., viral disease, myocarditis, end-stage HCM). Usually, diastolic dysfunction from ventricular stiffness is the major physiologic alteration, but this syndrome is quite diverse and systolic dysfunction may predominate. RCM has also been referred to as *intermediate cardiomyopathy (ICM)*.

Diagnosis and Treatment

Diagnostic tests are similar to HCM. Echocardiography helps define whether the disease has characteristics that are closer to HCM or DCM. Severe left atrial (+/− right atrial) enlargement is classic. The atrial enlargement often appears significantly greater than changes in the respective ventricle. Treatment usually is the same as that used for HCM (diastolic dysfunction). However, if systolic dysfunction is present, treatment may be more similar to DCM (see later). Atrial fibrillation, ventricular arrhythmias, and thrombosis are more common in RCM/ICM. Pleural effusions can be especially problematic. Prognosis tends to be poor, with most patients only surviving a few months after diagnosis. However, 1 to 2 years survival times have been noted.

Dilated Cardiomyopathy

Cause and Pathophysiology

In the late 1980s, DCM was associated with taurine deficient diets in cats. Today, DCM is uncommonly recognized in cats, and may or may not be a result of taurine deficiency. DCM may be secondary to other processes such as toxicity, myocarditis, or possibly an inherited trait. As with the dog, a decline in cardiac output (from pump failure) is the initial hemodynamic abnormality, but exercise intolerance may be difficult to identify in the cat. Thus most feline patients present in CHF (pulmonary edema +/− pleural effusion). The gallop sound heard in this disorder is that of rapid ventricular filling (S_3).

Treatment

Systolic dysfunction is the major hemodynamic pathology. Treatment principles are similar to DCM in the dog. A whole blood taurine level should be obtained in cats, particularly if the dietary history is questionable. Anticoagulant therapy is used as in HCM and RCM.

Myocarditis

Viral myocarditis (such as coronavirus) is difficult to document, although some have speculated that

RCM may be the result of a viral insult. Bacterial endocarditis or myocarditis is rare in cats. Siamese breeds
have been reported to have an increased incidence.
Inflammatory conditions such as neoplastic disease
(e.g., lymphoma, mesothelioma) or infectious conditions (e.g., *Toxoplasma* sp.) are occasionally recognized.
Patients with myocarditis often present with DCM-like
disease. Arrhythmias are common with any type of
myocarditis.

Thromboembolic Disease

Thromboembolic disease can be a complication secondary to any cardiac disorder in the cat. HCM and RCM are
the most frequently diagnosed diseases. The thrombus
usually forms within the left atrium, particularly the atrial appendage. Clot formation is thought to be due to
blood statis within the enlarged left atrium; however,
platelet dysfunction, amino acid abnormalities, and
coagulation factor alterations have also been demonstrated in some cats with cardiac disease. The most common location for thrombi at presentation is the
trifurcation of the distal aorta (saddle thrombus), followed by the right forelimb (right brachial artery). A
residual thrombus may or may not be visualized in the
left atrium per echocardiography on presentation.
Many cats will walk again with supportive care and anticoagulant therapy. However, the prognosis is very guard-

ed owing to the severity of cardiac disease and the extension of the thrombi (i.e., renal arteries). Those cats that survive an initial thrombolic episode are thought to be at increased risk for future episodes.

$\underline{7}$

Acquired Valvular Diseases

Degenerative Valvular Disease

Cause

Genetic factors are likely responsible for myxomatous degeneration of the valves.

The breeds that are commonly affected are the Poodle, Miniature Schnauzer, Chihuahua, Cocker Spaniel, terriers, and many small breeds of dogs. An incidence of greater than 50% has been noted in Cavalier King Charles Spaniels after 4 years of age.

Pathophysiology

The mitral valve is most commonly affected; however, the tricuspid valve may be affected in addition to or sometimes independent from the mitral. The aortic and pulmonic valves are rarely involved. Dilation (eccentric hypertrophy) of the related ventricle, atrium, and valve annulus results from the insufficient valve. Volume overload and dilation eventually leads to increased filling pressure and "back-up" behind the affected chambers. When pulmonary edema, pleural effusion, or ascites results from vascular congestion, congestive heart failure is present.

Clinical Presentation

Murmurs indicative of valvular disease are found at the left apex (mitral regurgitation [MR]) or at the right apex (tricuspid regurgitation [TR]). The murmurs of atrioventricular (AV) valve insufficiency are typically holosystolic and have a flat or plateau sound characteristic. Coughing and respiratory distress from pulmonary edema (left-sided congestive heart failure [CHF]) or pleural effusion, ascites, and jugular pulsations (right-sided CHF) may be initial problems. Fever or severe systemic illness and the finding of a new murmur may alert the clinician to the possibility of endocarditis.

Diagnosis

THORACIC RADIOGRAPH Left atrial and ventricular enlargement is documented with MR and is usually progressive over years. Pulmonary venous congestion and interstitial edema (typically hilar and caudodorsal) are noted when left-sided heart failure ensues. Right-sided abnormalities are noted with tricuspid insufficiency, that is, enlargement of the chambers of the right side of the heart, caudal vena cava, hepatomegaly, with or without pleural effusion and ascites.

ELECTROCARDIOGRAPHY Left atrial and ventricular enlargement patterns may be noted, but often the electrocardiogram (ECG) is normal in mild-to-moderate disease. Heart rate and rhythm are often normal, but ventricular and especially supraventricular arrhythmias can be noted. Atrial fibrillation may occur in advanced disease with severe left atrial enlargement. Rhythm abnormalities may be associated with weakness or syncope and often cause decompensation or acute onset of CHF.

ECHOCARDIOGRAPHY Echocardiography confirms valvular deformity (nodular, thickened), insufficiency and associated chamber enlargements. Indices of contractility are usually normal (in contrast to dilated cardiomyopathy [DCM]). However, with long-standing disease, the heart's ability to hypertrophy can be overcome by extreme dilation and systolic performance may decline.

Therapy

Angiotensin-converting enzyme inhibitors (ACEis) and diuretics are the mainstays of therapy for diseases of volume overload (see Chapter 4). Digoxin is not always needed unless systolic dysfunction is documented or significant supraventricular arrhythmias are noted.

Patient Monitoring

Monitor progression of valvular insufficiency and chamber enlargements (thoracic radiographs at minimum), renal enzymes, electrolytes, and for the occurrence of CHF. Medication adjustments are typically required with time as the disease progresses.

PROGNOSIS Survival time varies from months to years. Some dogs live more than 3 to 4 years past initial heart failure with attentive management.

Special Considerations

Treatment of dogs without heart failure is controversial. There has been some suggestion that prophylactic use of an ACEi may beneficial to reduce severity of disease progression. However, the data are conflicitng. If treatment is elected, it would likely be most practical in patients with significant chamber enlargement (volume overload). Weight reduction and modest sodium restriction may be implemented in these asymptomatic patients.

Infective Endocarditis

Definition

Infection of the heart valves and endocardial tissues with bacteria is more commonly reported in dogs than in cats.

Cause

Infection usually arises elsewhere in the body (skin, gastrointestinal tract, urinary system) and infects the valves via bacteremia (Box 7-1). Valvular pathology (endocardiosis, dysplasia) predisposes the leaflet to infection. An increased incidence of bacterial endocarditis is noted for dogs with subaortic stenosis.

Pathophysiology

The mitral and aortic valves are most commonly affected in small animal species. Infection causes further deformity and insufficiency of the valve (Figure 7-1). Left ventricular volume overload occurs, and left-sided

---

Box 7-1.   Organisms Isolated in Infective Endocarditis

Most Common
Staphylococcus sp.
Streptococcus sp.
Escherichia coli

Less Common
Pasturella sp.
Pseudomonas sp.
Corynebacterium sp.
Erysipelothrix sp.

---

congestive heart failure may ensue. Symptoms of CHF may appear suddenly in patients with ruptured chordae tendineae and severe valve destruction. Fragments of the vegetative lesion (with or without bacteria) may break off and embolize other organ systems. Circulating immune complexes contribute to the disease state and are responsible for immune-mediated reactions such as polyarthropathy or glomerulonephritis.

Clinical Presentation

Large breed male dogs appear predisposed. Subaortic stenosis (SAS) is a known risk factor. Patients may present with "new" murmurs of mitral regurgitation or aortic insufficiency. Respiratory symptoms (congestive failure) may or may not be present. Nonspecific signs of lethargy,

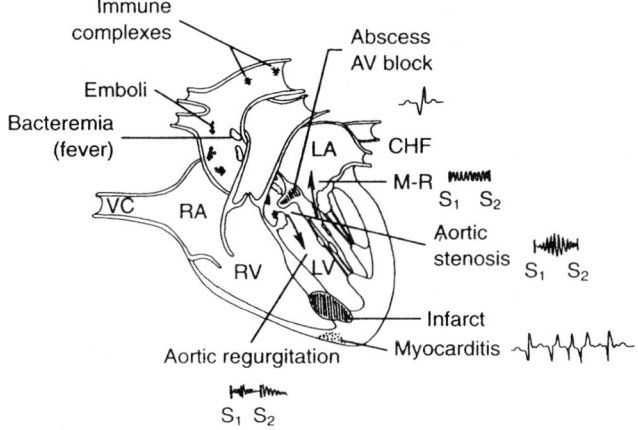

Figure 7-1. Summary of pathophysiologic processes in bacterial endocarditis. (*From Bongura JD (ed):* Saunders manual of small animal practice, *ed 2, Philadelphia, 2000, WB Saunders.*)

weight loss, and elusive fever are common. The dogs may have a history or obvious signs of lameness (polyarthropathy). The symptoms may be vague, wax and wane, and include multiple organs systems, giving this syndrome the nickname "the great imitator."

Diagnosis

THORACIC RADIOGRAPHS Radiographs correlate to underlying valvular pathology, that is, left atrial and ventricular enlargement for mitral valve involvement, with or without pulmonary edema (left-sided CHF).

ELECTROCARDIOGRAPHY Extension of infection or inflammation into the AV node may cause various degrees of heart block. Ventricular arrhythmias are common (myocardial inflammation).

ECHOCARDIOGRAPHY Volume overload and dilation of the affected chambers are noted. Irregular vegetative lesions and valve distortions are identified in chronic or severe disease. However, with acute or subacute endocarditis, minimal anatomic changes may be recognized. Systolic function may be impaired in some patients (e.g., those with myocarditis).

Therapy

Blood and urine cultures are indicated. Antibiotics should be based on results and sensitivity testing. While awaiting culture results, a broad-spectrum combination such as a cephalosporin or penicillin-derivative with an aminoglycoside or enrofloxacin is typically chosen. Antibacterial therapy should be administered intravenously for the first 3 to 5 days to obtain adequate blood levels. Oral medications should be continued for 4 to 6 weeks. Antiarrhythmic and heart failure therapies are often needed.

Prognosis

The long-term prognosis is guarded to poor, but aggressive therapy may be successful in some individuals. Congestive heart failure, sepsis, renal failure, and fatal embolism are usual causes of death.

8

Common Congenital Anomalies

Arteriovenous Shunts

Patent Ductus Arteriosis

DEFINITION AND CAUSE The ductus arteriosis (functional in fetal circulation) normally closes shortly after birth. In animals with inherited (polygenic trait) patent ductus arteriosus (PDA), the ductal wall is abnormal and closure does not occur.

PATHOPHYSIOLOGY (FIGURE 8-1) Blood shunts from the high-pressure aorta to the lower pressure pulmonary

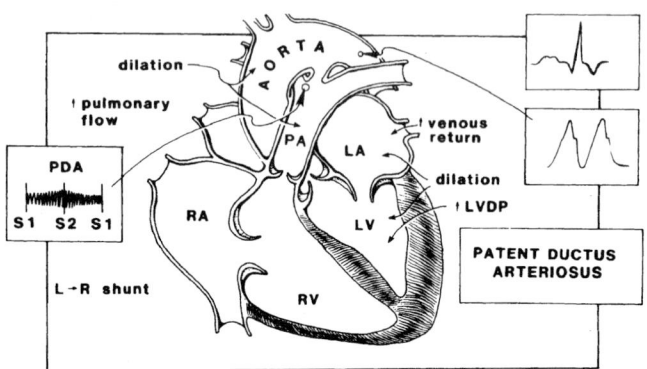

Figure 8-1. A schematic of the pathophysiology in PDA. See text for details. (*From Bonagura JD(ed):* Cardiology, *New York, 1987, Churchill Livingstone.*)

artery during the entire cardiac cycle. This left-to-right shunting of blood causes a volume overload of the pulmonary vessels, the left atrium, and the left ventricle. The volume of shunting is directly related to the diameter of the ductus and the pressure difference between the two circulations.

CLINICAL PRESENTATION

Signalment The condition occurs more often in females (three times greater than males). Bichon Frise, Maltese, Pomeranian, Shetland Sheepdog, English Springer Spaniel, Keeshond, Poodle (toy and miniature),

Yorkshire terrier, Collie, and German shepherds are overrepresented. PDA is the most common congenital anomaly diagnosed in dogs.

CLINICAL EXAMINATION A *continuous murmur* heard high at the left heart base (over the ductus) is characteristic. Typically, a *precordial thrill* is palpated in the same area. *Hyperkinetic arterial pulses* are often appreciated owing to the widened pulse pressure (difference between systolic and diastolic). The continual runoff of blood from the arterial system through the ductus results in a lowered diastolic pressure. Left-sided congestive heart failure may or may not be present (tachypnea, coughing with or without pulmonary crackles).

DIAGNOSIS
Thoracic Radiographs Typical radiographic findings include, pulmonary overcirculation (enlarged arteries and veins); left atrial, auricular, and ventricular enlargement; main pulmonary artery bulge (dorsoventral [DV] projection); and descending aortic dilatation, that is, "ductus bump" (DV projection). Pulmonary edema may be present (~50% of cases).

Electrocardiogram Left ventricular enlargement pattern (tall R wave, with or without wide QRS), left atrial enlargement pattern (wide P wave) are common findings. Ventricular or supraventricular arrhythmias may be seen in chronic or severe cases. Not all cases demonstrate electrocardiographic (ECG) abnormalities.

Echocardiography Echocardiography confirms left atrial, auricular and ventricular enlargement (eccentric hypertrophy) and dilation of the main pulmonary artery. The ductus is usually difficult to visualize on the two-dimensional examination, but continuous flow (using color Doppler) in the main pulmonary artery is readily documented. Mitral valve regurgitation is often present owing to the geometric changes in the valve annulus as the left side of the heart enlarges. Estimates of systolic function may be abnormal in some severe or chronic cases (cardiomyopathy of volume overload).

THERAPY Occlusion of the ductus is the treatment of choice. Presently, two methods are used to accomplish this goal. Closure of the PDA is most often accomplished by surgical ligation of the vessel. Some (specialized) practices may deploy thrombogenic coils into the ductus through the femoral artery to cause embolization. Surgery is successful in more than 90% of cases. Fatal hemorrhage and cardiac arrest from pulmonary edema or arrhythmias are the most serious complications. Heart failure should *always* be treated (if present) before any anesthetic procedure. Furosemide and angiotensin-converting enzyme inhibitors (ACEis) are most commonly used.

PROGNOSIS If the condition is left untreated, 50% to 64% of patients with PDA will die within the first year. Prognosis is excellent with successful ductal occlusion; normal life span is expected. Heart failure usually resolves, and medications may be discontinued. Even patients with marginal systolic function (cardiomyopathy of chronic volume overload) may lead normal lives. Medications may or may not be permanently needed in this group.

Ventricular Septal Defect

DEFINITION AND CAUSE In ventricular septal defect (VSD), a portion of the septum is missing, resulting in an intracardiac arteriovenous shunt. The majority of VSDs are located in the membranous portion of the interventricular septum, just below the aortic valve on the left side to underneath the septal tricuspid leaflet on the right. The defect may be inherited in some breeds.

PATHOPHYSIOLOGY The magnitude of blood shunting depends on the size of the defect and the pressure difference between the two ventricles (Figure 8-2). Because left ventricular systolic pressures are higher than right ventricular systolic pressures, the shunt is typically left to right. Owing to the location of the defect, volume overload of the right ventricular outflow or main pulmonary artery, pulmonary vessels, and chambers of

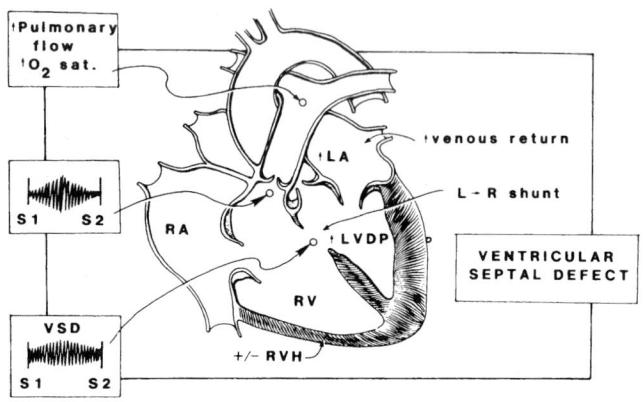

Figure 8-2. A schematic of the pathophysiology of VSD. See text for details. (*From Bonagura JD(ed): Cardiology, New York, 1987, Churchill Livingstone.*)

the left side of the heart is the result. Some very large defects may lead to right ventricular (RV) volume and pressure overload (eccentric and concentric hypertrophy) as more of the RV chamber is affected by the extra volume.

CLINICAL PRESENTATION

Signalment VSD is the most common congenital defect found in cats (no known breed predilection). Springer Spaniel, English Bulldog, and Keeshond breeds have increased incidence of VSD (possibly inherited).

Clinical Examination A holosystolic crescendo-decrescendo (ejection) murmur is heard best at the right sternal border. A precordial thrill may be present in the same location. Occasionally, a diastolic murmur (soft decrescendo) of aortic insufficiency is heard at the left heart base (loss of aortic root support). In some animals with large shunts, the murmur of relative pulmonic stenosis may be auscultated as a systolic ejection murmur at the left base. Relative stenosis means that a higher volume of blood is moving through an anatomically normal pulmonic valve at a higher velocity. Left-sided congestive heart failure (CHF) may or may not be present.

DIAGNOSIS
Thoracic Radiographs The pulmonary vessels appear overcirculated, and a bulge in the main pulmonary artery may be present (larger shunts). Left atrial, auricular, and ventricular enlargement is usually noted. Pulmonary edema may or may not be present. Right heart enlargement patterns may be seen if the defect is large.

Electrocardiogram The ECG may be normal or reveal left ventricular enlargement, with or without left atrial enlargement patterns.

Echocardiography Left atrial and ventricular dilation from volume overload are confirmed. The pulmonary artery may appear prominent. Color Doppler demonstrates the defect in the typical high septal location. Spectral Doppler can be used to assess the magnitude of the shunt. The size of shunt is directly related to the velocity of blood flow through the defect. Small defects maintain a relatively normal pressure difference between the two ventricles and exhibit very high velocity flows whereas large defects allow ventricular pressures to equilibrate, resulting in lower flow velocities.

TREATMENT Defects in the typical location are not often feasible to approach for primary intracardiac surgical closure. Small defects require no intervention, whereas defects with a flow velocity of 4 m/s or less (≤64 mm Hg pressure difference between the ventricles) may benefit from a *pulmonary artery banding procedure.* This technique serves to raise the right ventricular systolic pressure, thus decreasing the left-to-right shunting volume. With a reduction in the shunting, the volume overload of the lungs and left heart is partially alleviated. Therapy for CHF may be warranted in some cases.

PROGNOSIS The prognosis depends on the size of the defect and the potential secondary consequences such as CHF and cardiomyopathy of chronic volume overload. Patients with small defects may live completely normal lives.

Eisenmenger's Physiology

DEFINITION AND CAUSE In some animals, pulmonary volume overload from the left-to-right shunt causes injury to the pulmonary vasculature and pulmonary hypertension. When pulmonary pressures exceed systemic pressures, reversal of the shunt to right-to-left occurs. This is referred to as *Eisenmenger's physiology.*

PATHOPHYSIOLOGY The pulmonary vascular histologic changes may include intimal and medial hypertrophy, and fibrosis. Pulmonary vascular pressures rise, and as a result, right ventricular pressures become elevated. The volume of left-to-right shunt reduces, and if right heart pressures become greater than systemic pressures, shunt reversal occurs. Right-to-left shunts caused by pulmonary hypertension result in the delivery of unoxygenated blood to the systemic circulation. Polycythemia and blood hyperviscosity (from hypoxemia) contribute to the patients' symptoms.

CLINICAL PRESENTATION
History Animals usually present with a history of lethargy, exercise intolerance, respiratory compromise with exertion, or syncope. A history of a murmur or previously diagnosed shunting defect may not be noted, because many of these patients are thought to reverse very early in life (the first few weeks or months).

Clinical Examination Often, no murmur is appreciated (lower velocity shunting and hyperviscosity with polycythemia). As in many cases of pulmonary hypertension, a loud or split S_2 may be auscultated owing to snapping of the pulmonary valve. A prominent right precordium may be palpated, and jugular venous distension and pulsations may be present to indicate high right heart filling pressures. Patients with shunt reversal may appear cyanotic only during exercise; thus mucous membrane evaluation may be initially deceiving. It is important to note that reversed intracardiac shunts (VSD, atrial septal defect [ASD]) manifest systemic cyanosis, whereas the reversed extracardiac shunt of PDA results in caudal cyanosis. In reversed PDA, the cranial part of the body receives normally oxygenated blood through the brachiocephalic trunk and left subclavian artery (before the ductus), whereas the caudal part of the body receives poorly oxygenated blood. This phenomenon is referred to as *differential cyanosis*. Oral mucous membranes may appear pink, whereas caudal membranes (prepuce, vulva) are cyanotic.

DIAGNOSIS

Thoracic Radiographs Radiographs may reveal similar findings to primary disease but often have predominantly right atrial, ventricular, and main pulmonary artery enlargement. The pulmonary vessels may appear tortuous but no longer appear overcirculated. Right-sided CHF may or may not be present.

Electrocardiography The ECG may be normal, or right-sided heart enlargement patterns may be noted (rightward mean electrical axis [MEA]; deep S waves in leads I, II, III and AVF).

Echocardiography Two-dimensional echocardiography may reveal the primary defect, particularly if it is intracardiac, but readily confirms right atrial enlargement, right ventricular hypertrophy, and main pulmonary artery enlargement. The PDA defect is not seen on routine echocardiography. Color Doppler and especially an ultrasound contrast study (bubble study) may be performed to detect right-to-left shunting of blood of reversed PDA.

TREATMENT Surgery is *contraindicated* in these patients. The pulmonary vascular changes are permanent. If the patent ductus is ligated in this case, increasing right heart pressure overload and failure will ensue when the pressure pop-off valve is closed. Therapeutic goals are exercise limitation and maintain a packed cell volume (PCV) ~60%. Periodic phlebotomy (approximately every 4 to 6 weeks) is suggested to minimize the symptoms related to polycythemia and hyperviscosity. A typical blood donor aliquot of 20 ml/kg is removed.

PROGNOSIS Some patients live 5 to 10 years with a reversed defect and appropriate monitoring. Longer-term prognosis is poor.

Outflow Obstruction

Pulmonic Stenosis

DEFINITION Pulmonic stenosis (PS) is a congenital anomaly that may include fusion of the pulmonary valve cusps, malformation of the valve apparatus (dysplasia), hypoplasia of the valve annulus, or a combination of these pathologies.

PATHOPHYSIOLOGY In addition, the defect may be at the valve level, just above (supravalvular stenosis) or just below (subvalvular muscular stenosis) the valve level. Right ventricular pressure overload and concentric hypertrophy result from systolic outflow obstruction. Severe right ventricular hypertrophy promotes ischemia and arrhythmias. Right-sided heart failure (pleural effusion, ascites) can sometimes be seen.

CLINICAL PRESENTATION
Signalment Beagle, Boxer, English bulldog (male has a higher incidence than the female), Mastiff, Samoyed, Schnauzer, and terrier breeds are predisposed.

History Murmurs may be found incidentally; however, many symptomatic patients present for evaluation of collapse (syncope). CHF is uncommon unless another defect such as tricuspid dysplasia is present.

Clinical Examination A systolic crescendo-decrescendo (ejection-type) murmur is typically present at the left heart base. A holosystolic murmur of tricuspid insufficiency may be auscultated at the right apex in some cases. A prominent right precordium may be palpable, and jugular pulsations may be present to indicate high right heart filling pressures.

DIAGNOSIS

Thoracic Radiographs Classically, a "reversed D" of right ventricular hypertrophy, right atrial enlargement, and pulmonary trunk bulge are noted on the dorsoventral view. The pulmonary vessels may appear normal or undercirculated.

Electrocardiography Right ventricular enlargement pattern (right axis deviation; deep S waves in leads I, II, III, AVF) may be present. Ventricular arrhythmias are not uncommon and may be responsible for syncope. Not all patients have ECG abnormalities.

Echocardiography Right ventricular hypertrophy with or without dilation are identified. The interventricular septum may appear flattened owing to the pressure over-load on the right and displacement of the septum to the left. Right atrial enlargement is noted, and tricuspid regurgitation may or may not be present. An immobile and thickened pulmonic valve can usually be seen. The velocity of blood flow (spectral Doppler) through the stenosis is directly related to the severity of the defect; the greater the velocity, the tighter the stenosis. The maximum velocity is used to calculate a pressure difference between the right ventricle and pulmonary artery. This information is also used to gauge treatment and prognosis.

TREATMENT Patients with mild pressure gradients of 50 mm Hg or less often do not need therapy. Treatment is usually indicated with pulmonic Doppler velocities of more than 5m/s (100 mm Hg pressure gradient across the stenosis). Transvenous balloon dilation of the pulmonic valve can be performed in many patients with good results. Patients that are not suitable candidates for balloon valvuloplasty (significant annular hypoplasia) or respond poorly to the procedure may benefit from a surgical intervention. There are several surgical techniques described to apply a patch graft (pericardial or synthetic) over the right ventricular outflow tract or to bypass the outflow tract with a conduit. The perioperative mortality rate may be as high as 25% with these more aggressive surgical techniques.

A beta blocker may be helpful in some animals alone or in conjunction with an interventional procedure to help relieve the effects of outflow obstruction, especially if significant infundibular hypertrophy is present. Right-sided CHF, if present, requires medical therapy with diuretics and an ACEi.

SPECIAL CONSIDERATIONS English bulldogs and Boxers diagnosed with PS should undergo cardiac catheterization for evaluation of an anomalous left coronary artery, which arises from the right coronary ostia and encircles the right ventricular outflow tract. These dogs present a dilemma for repair because the anomalous artery may be severed during valvuloplasty or surgery. Placing an artificial conduit between the right ventricle and pulmonary artery may be the best option, particularly if the patient's response to medical therapy is incomplete.

PROGNOSIS The prognosis of animals with PS varies with severity of disease. Mild-to-moderate PS patients may live normal lives, whereas severely affected animals usually die within 3 years of diagnosis. Sudden death (presumably due to arrhythmia) is common. Animals demonstrating tricuspid dysplasia or severe tricuspid regurgitation, CHF, or atrial fibrillation have a considerably worse prognosis.

Subaortic Stenosis

DEFINITION AND CAUSE In subaortic stenosis (SAS), a fibrous ring or band encircles the left ventricular outflow tract below the aortic valve and obstructs ventricular emptying. This anomaly may be inheritable as an autosomal dominant trait.

PATHOPHYSIOLOGY Concentric left ventricular hypertrophy results in myocardial ischemia and fibrosis as the myocardium outgrows its blood supply (Figure 8-3). Ventricular arrhythmias are especially common with moderate to severe disease. As with PS, SAS disease severity can vary considerably among patients. True *aortic* stenosis is rare in the dog.

CLINICAL PRESENTATION
Signalment Newfoundland, Golden Retriever, Boxer, Rottweiler, German Shepherd, English Bulldog, Great Dane, and other large or sporting breeds are overrepresented. SAS is the second most common congenital anomaly found in dogs.

Clinical Examination A systolic crescendo-decrescendo (ejection-type) murmur is heard best over the low left heart base (below the aortic valve area). A precordial thrill may be present in the same location. The murmur may radiate to the right base (root of the ascending aorta), up the carotid arteries, and up to the calvarium. In moderate-to-severe SAS, weak and late rising femoral pulses may be noted (when compared with the precordium). Occasionally, the diastolic murmur of con-

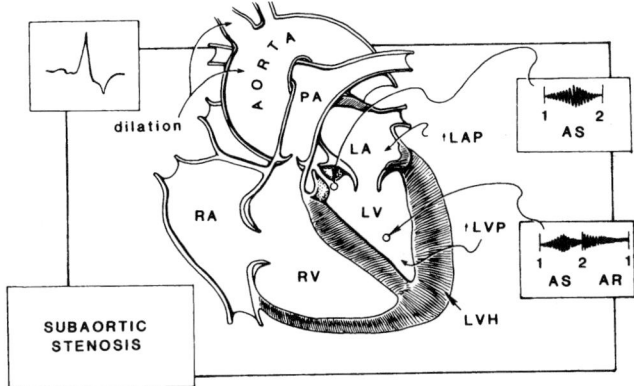

Figure 8-3. A schematic of the pathophysiology of SAS. See text for details. (*From Bonagura JD(ed):* Cardiology, *New York, 1987, Churchill Livingstone.*)

current aortic regurgitation may be heard at the left heart base.

DIAGNOSIS

Thoracic Radiographs Left-sided cardiomegaly may be prominent, but normal radiographic appearance of the heart is noted in some (particularly young) animals. A widened cranial cardiac margin may be present owing to dilation of the ascending aorta (poststenotic dilation).

Electrocardiography The ECG may be normal or may indicate left ventricular enlargement with or without left axis deviation. Ventricular arrhythmias are common especially in severe and long-standing cases.

Echocardiography Left ventricular hypertrophy and left atrial enlargement are typical. The subendocardial regions of the left ventricle may appear bright compared with other portions of the myocardium. This likely represents fibrotic change from chronic ischemia. The subaortic ridge or ring can usually be seen in moderate-to-severe cases. Turbulence in the left ventricular outflow tract and ascending aorta is noted, and aortic and mitral regurgitation may be appreciated with color Doppler. Spectral Doppler is needed to assess the severity of the disease. Outflow tract velocities greater than 5.6 m/s (125 mm Hg pressure gradient) are considered severe disease.

TREATMENT Medical therapy is the treatment of choice at this time. Beta blockers are indicated in moderate-to-severe cases to reduce outflow obstruction, increase diastolic filling times, and promote myocardial perfusion. They may also be helpful in minimizing arrhythmias. Balloon valvuloplasty may temporarily help some dogs (particularly with rare aortic stenosis [AS]), but many will develop restenosis with time. Various surgical techniques have been shown to reduce outflow obstruction, but the incidence of sudden death and survival times are not significantly altered as compared with medical therapy alone.

PROGNOSIS Approximately 50% of severely affected dogs (125 mm Hg pressure gradient) will die suddenly before 3 years of age. It is unknown whether medical therapy will alter survival times. CHF may develop later in some animals. Patients with SAS appear to be at increased risk for infective endocarditis.

Atrioventricular Valve Malformation

Mitral Dysplasia

DEFINITION AND PATHOPHYSIOLOGY Many types of congenital malformations of the mitral valve apparatus have been identified. Valvular regurgitation is the predominant finding. However, mitral stenosis may be present in some cases. Volume overload of the left atrium and ventricle causes dilation (eccentric hypertrophy) of both chambers. Left-sided CHF (pulmonary edema) results from increased left heart filling pressures and pulmonary venous hypertension.

CLINICAL PRESENTATION
Signalment Males are more commonly affected than females. Great Dane, Bull Terrier, German Shepherd,

Newfoundland, Mastiff, and other large or giant breeds are overrepresented. Mitral dysplasia is the second most common congenital anomaly in cats.

Clinical Examination A holosystolic (plateau-type) heart murmur is best heard over the left apex. Pulmonary crackles and harsh noises may be auscultated if left-sided CHF is present. Patients with chronic left-sided CHF may develop significant pulmonary arterial hypertension and right-sided CHF as well.

DIAGNOSIS
Thoracic Radiographs Left-sided cardiomegaly, especially of the atrium, is classically present. Enlarged pulmonary veins and interstitial opacities (i.e., hilar regions) may be noted if CHF has occurred.

Electrocardiography Widened P waves of left atrial enlargement are commonly found in severely affected animals. Left ventricular enlargement patterns and supraventricular arrhythmias (atrial premature beats or atrial fibrillation) may be seen.

Echocardiography Echocardiography confirms left atrial and ventricular dilation. Specific mitral valve defects can be identified. Doppler demonstrates mitral valve insufficiency with or without restriction to filling (if stenosis is present).

TREATMENT Treatment is the same as for acquired mitral valve disease. Diuretics (i.e., furosemide) and ACEi (i.e., enalapril) are used to control pulmonary edema and excess fluid volume retention. Digoxin may be indicated in some patients with supraventricular arrhythmias or if systolic dysfunction has developed from chronic or severe volume overload. Surgical valve reconstruction or replacement is available at a few veterinary medical centers.

PROGNOSIS The prognosis is generally poor with severe disease and refractory CHF.

Tricuspid Dysplasia

DEFINITION AND PATHOPHYSIOLOGY Several types of congenital malformations of the tricuspid valve are noted, including displacement of the valve apparatus into the ventricle (Ebstein's anomaly). Commonly, there is thickening of the valve leaflets, underdevelopment of the chordae and papillary muscles, and incomplete separation of the medial valve from the septal wall. The hemodynamic consequences are due to tricuspid regurgitation (stenosis is rare). Volume overload of the right atrium and ventricle causes dilation (eccentric hypertrophy) of both chambers. This defect is sometimes associated with a supraventricular tachyarrhythmia called *Wolff-Parkinson-White (WPW) syndrome*. This arrhythmia causes ventricular preexcitation through a fast accessory path and may be responsible for syncope in some pets.

CLINICAL PRESENTATION

Signalment Males are more commonly affected than females. Labrador Retriever (may be familial), German Shepherd, Great Dane, Weimaraner, Old English Sheepdog, Borzoi, Irish Setter, Newfoundland, Shih Tzu, and Boxer breeds are more frequently reported.

Clinical Examination A holosystolic (plateau-type) murmur is heard best over the right apex. Pleural fluid may be appreciated as muffled heart and lung sounds ventrally if congestive right heart failure is present. Abdominal distension and ballotable fluid may also be noted if right-sided CHF has occurred. Jugular distension and pulsations indicate elevated right heart filling pressures.

DIAGNOSIS

Thoracic Radiographs Right atrial, ventricular, and caudal vena caval enlargement are classic findings. The heart often appears somewhat globoid, but the point of the normal left ventricular apex may be preserved. Pleural effusion, ascites, or hepatomegaly may be noted.

Electrocardiography Right atrial (tall P wave) and ventricular (deep S waves) enlargement patterns may be seen. Atrial fibrillation is common with severe right atrial

(RA) enlargement. Paroxysmal supraventricular tachy-cardia (WPW-like syndrome) may be identified, particularly on a Holter recording of a syncopal patient.

Echocardiography Echocardiography confirms RA and RV dilation. Specific tricuspid valve defects can be seen. Color flow Doppler demonstrates severe tricuspid insufficiency.

TREATMENT Medical management of right-sided CHF may be needed. Diuretics and ACEi are used, as in other volume overload diseases. Digoxin (and other antiarrhythmic drugs) may be indicated if supraventricular arrhythmias are documented. Surgical valve reconstruction or replacement is available at a few veterinary medical centers.

PROGNOSIS The prognosis depends on the severity of the disease. Many dogs live normal spans with significant tricuspid dysplasia. Dogs with signs of CHF before 1 year of age usually have a poor prognosis.

Cyanotic Heart Disease

Tetralogy of Fallot

DEFINITION AND PATHOPHYSIOLOGY This anomaly consists of VSD (usually large), PS, RV hypertrophy, and rightward displacement of the aorta over the VSD (straddling the two ventricles). With the elevated RV pressures from PS and systemic or aortic resistance, blood shunts from the right ventricle to the aorta. The degree of RV-to-aortic shunting depends upon the magnitude of the PS and VSD (and therefore RV pressure). Some animals experience significant clinical right-to-left shunting primarily with exercise (increases pulmonary and thus RV pressures).

CLINICAL PRESENTATION

Signalment The Keeshond (polygenic inheritance) and English Bulldog have shown an increased incidence.

Clinical Examination Murmurs of PS and VSD may be auscultated. However, many animals have no audible murmur owing to the hyperviscosity syndrome resulting from significant hypoxia and polycythemia. Jugular pulsations may be present. Cyanosis may be present at rest or only after exercise.

DIAGNOSIS

Thoracic Radiographs Cardiomegaly is variable on radiographs. Pulmonary vessels may appear small (PS), or pulmonary vascularity may appear increased (compensatory increase in bronchial arteries). The malpositioned aorta may bulge cranially on the lateral view.

Electrocardiography The ECG may reveal right-sided heart enlargement patterns.

Echocardiography Echocardiography demonstrates the defects. Doppler and contrast studies can reveal the degree of right to left shunting and assess severity of the anomaly.

TREATMENT Periodic phlebotomy to maintain the PCV about 60% is usually necessary for severely affected patients. Beta blockers may be useful in some patients to reduce right ventricular outflow obstruction and promote myocardial perfusion. Definitive repair requires open-heart surgery (available at a few veterinary institutions). Palliative surgical procedures creating a left-to-right shunt to increase blood flow to the lungs have been used successfully. These procedures may increase overall patient oxygenation by allowing for more mixing of oxygenated blood. Anastomosis of the left subclavian artery to the pulmonary artery (Blalock's anastomosis) or side-to-side anastomosis of the aorta to the pulmonary artery (Potts' anastomosis) has been performed to create left-to-right shunting.

PROGNOSIS The prognosis depends on the severity of the disease and the success of the treatment. Some patients may live 4 to 7 years with mild disease and conservative therapies.

Vascular Ring Anomalies

Definition and Pathophysiology

The most commonly reported thoracic vascular anomaly (after PDA) is persistent right aortic arch (PRAA). Other malformations of the embryonic arches may occur alone or in conjunction with PRAA. Retention of the right aortic arch versus the normal left arch causes entrapment of the esophagus between the arch (right and dorsal), the ligamentum arteriosum (left), and the heart base (ventrally). Dilatation of the esophagus, cranial to the heart base, results from the entrapment.

Presentation and Diagnosis

German Shepherds, Great Danes, and Irish Setters appear predisposed to this condition. Regurgitation and stunted growth are the typical clinical signs and are usually noted soon after weaning. Thoracic radiographs (and esophagram) reveal a dilated esophagus cranial to the heart base.

Treatment and Prognosis

Therapy involves surgical resection of the ligamentum arteriosum to alleviate the stricture. The prognosis is variable for resolution of regurgitation because permanent esophageal dilatation and dysmotility are common. Some patients have minimal clinical signs after surgery (maintaining upright feedings), whereas others have significant regurgitation or episodes of aspiration pneumonia.

9

Pericardial Diseases

Pericardial Effusion

Definition

Pericardial effusions are a collection of fluid within the pericardial space. The effusions may be exudates, transudates, or hemorrhagic fluids.

Cause

The most common cause of pericardial effusions, particularly *hemorrhagic* effusions, is neoplasia. Benign pericardial effusion often identified in young, middle-age large breed dogs is also hemorrhagic (second most common hemorrhagic effusion). Occasionally, left atrial rupture (from severe left atrial enlargement), coagulopathies (e.g., rodenticide toxicosis), and trauma are causes of pericardial hemorrhage. *Transudative* effusions may be seen with congestive heart failure (CHF), hypoalbuminemia, or some systemic vasculopathies. In these cases, the effusion volume is usually small. *Exudates* are uncommon and are typically secondary a systemic infectious process such as septicemia, fungal infections, and feline infectious peritonitis (FIP) virus.

Pathophysiology

Fluid accumulating in the pericardial space progressively increases intrapericardial pressures. When intrapericardial pressures exceed right heart (diastolic) filling pressures, external compression of the right side of the heart (especially atrium) results (see Figure 9-1). Cardiac filling is impaired, and systemic venous pressures progressively increase, causing signs of right-sided CHF. As cardiac filling is impaired, forward output eventually falls, leading to systemic hypotension and weakness. This phenomenon is referred to as *cardiac tamponade*.

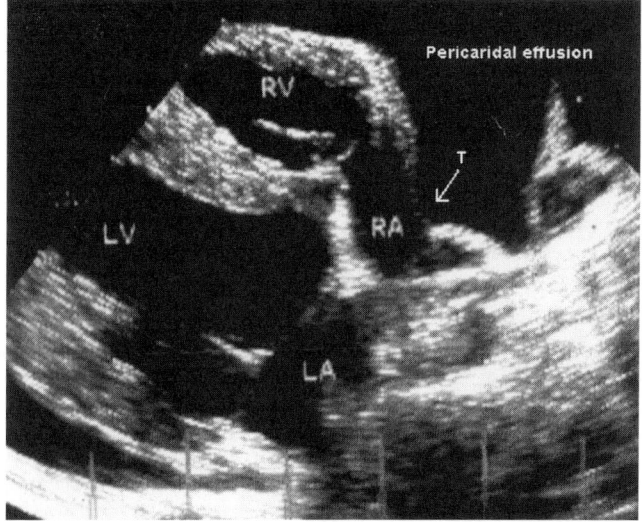

Figure 9-1. An echocardiogram in a German Shepherd dog with pericardial effusion. Note the anechoic space around the heart (effusion) and the collapse of the right atrial wall. T, Echo tamponade.

Clinical Presentation

Signs of right-sided heart failure (pleural and abdominal effusions, jugular distension and pulsations) predominate. Most patients have weak peripheral pulses, diminished precordium, and muffled heart sounds on examination. A palpable decrease in pulse strength during inspiration (pulsus paradoxus) is a classic finding in patients with pericardial effusion. Many pets will appear amazingly healthy if the effusion has developed slowly (allowing pericardial stretch and pet compensation). Others will appear to be very weak, lethargic, or in circulatory shock.

Diagnosis

THORACIC RADIOGRAPHS Classically, chest radiographs demonstrate a very large and globoid cardiac silhouette. The normal contours of the heart are lost in the circumferential effusion. Pleural effusion (right-sided CHF), pulmonary edema (left-sided CHF), and caudal vena cava distension are commonly present.

ELECTROCARDIOGRAPHY Small voltage QRS complexes and electrical alternans (alternating change in the R amplitude) are consistent with pericardial effusion but are not found in every case.

ECHOCARDIOGRAPHY Echocardiography is the most sensitive test for detecting even small pericardial effusions (Figure 9-1). An anechoic space between the heart and the hyperechoic pericardium is noted. The fluid is helpful to visualize tumors.

Therapy

The *only therapy* to alleviate signs of pericardial effusion and cardiac tamponade is *pericardiocentesis*. Diuretics will not mobilize the effusion and only serve to deplete the vascular volume, further exacerbating hypotension. Pericardiocentesis is usually performed from the patient's right side. This approach minimizes trauma to the lungs (cardiac notch) and laceration of a coronary vessel (more prominent on the left). A pericardiotomy or a pericardial window (created surgically or by balloon dilation) may be indicated in patients with benign pericardial effusion or slow growing tumors to alleviate signs of tamponade.

Prognosis

Prognosis depends upon the etiology of the effusion.

NEOPLASIA Hemangiosarcoma, the most common cause of pericardial effusion in the dog, carries a poor prognosis owing to rapid tumor metastasis. Pericardectomy is not feasible in this group owing to rapid disease progression and the potential for severe hemorrhage into the chest cavity. Chemotherapy can sometimes retard tumor growth, decrease effusion formation, and palliate clinical signs. Patients with slow-growing chemodectomas may have better survival times (1+ years) with pericardectomy or creation of a pericardial window.

These tumors are locally invasive but do not commonly metastasize. Alleviating the cardiac tamponade may afford good quality of life for some time.

INFECTIOUS Animals with infectious pericarditis generally require surgery (thoracotomy, pericardectomy, and chest drains) or minimally, drain placement into the pericardium. The prognosis depends on success of treatment of the underlying disease, but it is generally considered guarded.

BENIGN Dogs with benign pericardial effusions may resolve after one or two drainage procedures. Corticosteroids have been suggested in this group to treat a suspected inflammatory condition. Pericardectomy or pericardial window placement may be needed in those in which effusions occur repeatedly. Prognosis is fair to good in this group.

Constrictive Pericardial Disease

Definition and Cause

The pericardium may become thickened and fibrotic, and adhere to the epicardium. The stiff pericardium may inhibit ventricular relaxation and filling during diastole. In some cases, a small amount of effusion is present in the pericardial space (constrictive-effusive pericarditis). The cause of constrictive pericarditis is usually not clear. Some have proposed that this condition may be the result of a viral insult or a chronic inflammatory (immune-mediated) process. In some patients, neoplasia (e.g., mesothelioma) or fungal disease (e.g., infection with *Coccidioides* sp.) is found as an underlying cause.

Clinical Presentation and Treatment

Clinical signs are similar to that of chronic pericardial effusion and tamponade. Thoracic radiographs do not reveal the large, globoid cardiac silhouette that is seen with classic pericardial effusion. Pericardectomy and biopsy of the pericardium are indicated.

Peritoneal Pericardial Diaphragmatic Hernia

A congenital malformation of the pericardium allows communication between the pericardium and the peritoneal space in peritoneal pericardial diaphragmatic hernia (PPDH). Abdominal organs such as intestines and liver may be displaced into the pericardial space. Animals may be symptomatic, but often, the diagnosis is made incidentally. Symptoms, if present, typically relate to the gastrointestinal tract. Repair is indicated only if clinical signs are evident. In asymptomatic (particularly older) pets, attempts at repair may cause significant trauma to the adhered organs.

10

Pulmonary Hypertension

Definition and Causes

Pulmonary hypertension (PH) is an increase in pulmonary vascular resistance caused by vasoconstriction, vascular obstruction, or vascular volume overload (Box 10-1). PH may be an acute or chronic condition. Pulmonary hypertension is typically a secondary phenomenon; thus, recognizing the existence of PH is not analogous to diagnosing the patient's underlying condition. It is recognized secondary to many pulmonary parenchymal and vascular disorders.

Box 10-1.   Causes of Pulmonary Hypertension

Acute pressure overload
Pulmonary thromboembolism
Acute respiratory distress syndrome
Acute hypoxic pneumonia
Extensive lung resection

Chronic pressure overload
Chronic airway diseases (bronchitis, bronchiectasis,
    emphysema)
Chronic parenchymal disorders (neoplasia, pulmonary
    eosinophilic granulomatosus)
Restrictive lung disease (pleural and pleural space disease)
Chronic pulmonary thrombosis
Heartworm disease
Congenital heart disease
Occasionally idiopathic

Pathophysiology

Elevations in pulmonary arterial pressure are accompanied by elevations in right ventricular (RV) afterload, preload, intraventricular pressure, and heart rate. As RV pressure rises, the interventricular septum shifts to the left, impairing left ventricular filling. A vicious circle may ensue in which additional increases in RV pressure promote RV dilation, thus worsening left ventricular (LV) filling (and output). These events further exacerbate myocardial ischemia and systemic hypotension. Right-sided heart failure (pleural effusion, ascites) can also occur.

Clinical Presentation

Symptoms are usually referable to the underlying disease process. Tachypnea, cough, and exercise intolerance (hypoxia and hypotension) are common. A sudden onset of respiratory distress may be noted if the cause of PH is an acute or an acute-on-chronic process. Jugular distension and pulsations suggest elevated right heart filling pressures. The precordial impulse may feel stronger on the right hemithorax (suggesting RV enlargement). Right-sided heart failure may be present (pleural effusion, ascites).

Auscultation may reveal tricuspid regurgitation (right cardiac apex), split S_2, or loud snappy S_2 (left heart base) and a right-sided gallop sound.

Diagnosis

History of predisposing factors combined with appropriate clinical signs may suggest the presence of PH. Thoracic radiographs and echocardiogram may reveal minimal abnormalities or may show the classic findings in Box 10-2. Right heart or pulmonary arterial catheterization can definitively document right heart and pulmonary arterial pressures.

Box 10-2.   Radiographic and Echocardiographic Findings
in Pulmonary Hypertension

Thoracic Radiographs
Enlargement of proximal pulmonary arteries
Attenuation of peripheral pulmonary vessels
Right atrial +/– ventricular enlargement
Mild pleural effusion
Pulmonary parenchymal opacities

Echocardiogram
Poorly contracting right ventricle
TR velocities can estimate RV systolic pressure/pulmonary
    arterial systolic pressure
Leftward displacement of the septum
Pulmonary artery dilation (pulmonic regurgitation can estimate
    diastolic pulmonary arterial pressures)
Thrombus or heartworms

TR, Tricuspid regurgitation; *RV*, right ventricular.

Treatment

OXYGEN Enhance arterial oxygen (O_2) saturation and
minimize oxygen demands (sedation, treat fever, venti-
late). One goal may be to keep arterial O_2 saturation
greater than 96% in an attempt to avoid confounding
hypoxic pulmonary vasoconstriction.

VASCULAR VOLUME Finding the patient's optimal circulating fluid volume can be challenging. Aggressive intra-

venous fluids may exacerbate right ventricular pressure overload and displace the interventricular septum, impairing left ventricular filling and output. If no benefit is noted to discrete fluid therapy, vasoactive drug therapy should be considered. Vasoactive drugs may be beneficial to increase right heart cardiac output (dobutamine, dopamine). Dopamine may also enhance renal perfusion in a patient who may be suffering from poor systemic output.

ARTERIAL DILATION Pulmonary arterial dilator therapy has received much attention, but specific therapy is not well established. Oxygen is the most potent arterial dilator for the pulmonary system. Calcium-channel blockers have been advocated as a pulmonary artery dilator, particularly in mild to moderate cases of PH. Inhaled nitric oxide is a potent pulmonary vasodilator, but it can be difficult to administer long-term to veterinary patients. Prostaglandin E_1 is under investigation in humans with PH. Treatment of underlying condition is of utmost importance.

Patient Monitoring

The patient's response to therapy is used to guide treatment. Respiratory rate and effort, serial blood gases or pulse oximetry, pulmonary, and systemic blood pressures, and thoracic radiographs are typical parameters to evaluate. Prognosis depends on the severity of the PH and the underlying condition.

Special Considerations in Pulmonary Hypertension

Heartworm Disease

DEFINITION AND CAUSE Heartworm disease is a unique cause of pulmonary arterial hypertension in veterinary patients. Canids are primarily the species affected, but some felids and mustelids can harbor the parasites. The parasites reside in the pulmonary arteries, resulting in villous intimal hypertrophy. Arterial fibrosis, thrombosis, and vasoconstriction contribute to the syndrome of pulmonary hypertension. The infective larvae are transmitted to the host by the mosquito. Heartworm disease has been diagnosed in all 50 states; however, it is prevalent along the eastern and gulf coasts, and the Mississippi River valley. Figure 10-1 depicts the life cycle of the heartworm.

PATHOPHYSIOLOGY In addition to the pathophysiology of PH, heartworm disease is associated with unique complications and inflammatory conditions. *Vena caval syndrome* is a condition of circulatory shock caused by a mass of heartworms that have migrated backward into the right side of the heart and cava, obstructing cardiac filling. Severe shearing and lysing of red blood cells is often simultaneously noted. Emergent removal of the obstructive worm mass is indicated. Other relatively common

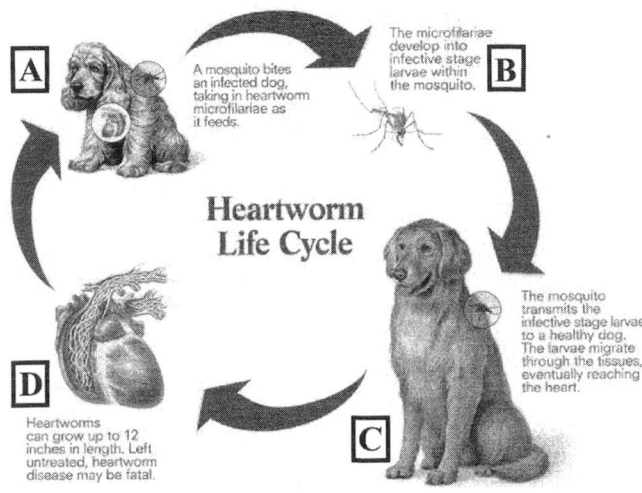

Figure 10.1. The life cycle of the heartworm (*Dirofilaria immitis*). **A,** The mosquito ingests the first stage larvae from an infected host. **B,** The larvae molt twice within the mosquito (L1 > L2 > L3). **C,** The L3 larvae enter the new host when the mosquito takes a blood meal. The larvae molt as they travel from the subcutis to the pulmonary vascular system. (L3 > L4 > L5). **D,** The young worms migrate to the caudal pulmonary arteries and mature into adults. It takes 5 to 6 months before the infection becomes patent (microfilaria are produced) in the new host. Reproduced with permission from Merial.

syndromes are *glomerulonephropathy* (antigen-antibody complex deposition) and *pulmonary eosinophilic granulomatosis* (hypersensitivity lung disease).

DIAGNOSIS The American Heartworm Society recommends adult heartworm antigen testing as the primary means of diagnosis. The antigen is from the female worm reproductive tract. There are several enzyme-linked immunoassay (ELISA) kits (Synbiotics, IDEXX), a hemaglutination test (Rhone-Merieux), and an immunochromatographic assay (Synbiotics). False-positive results are usually the result of a technical error, whereas false-negative results may be found with low worm burdens, immature female infection, all-male infection, or technical error. Concentration tests (millipore filter, Modified Knott's tests) may be used to detect microfilariae, particularly in those receiving diethylcarbamazine as a heartworm preventive (or no preventive). However, concentration tests are not recommended for routine screening owing to the wide fluctuations in circulating microfilariae or the lack of microfilariae present in an individual. Clinical presentation, and radiographic and echocardiographic findings are similar to other causes of PH. Classically, heartworm disease is associated with tortuous pulmonary arteries, particularly noted in the caudal lobar arteries on the dorsoventral radiograph.

TREATMENT All patients should have a thorough physical examination, radiographs, and metabolic evaluation before therapy with an adulticide (Table 10-1 and Boxes 10-3 and 10-4). Complications of therapy may be related

Table 10-1. Classification of Heartworm Disease Severity in Dogs

Class	Clinical signs	Radiographic signs	Laboratory abnormalities
1 (mild)	None; or occasional cough, fatigue or mild loss of body condition	None	None
2 (moderate)	None; or occasional cough, fatigue or moderate loss of body condition	Right ventricular enlargement ± some pulmonary artery enlargement; ± perivascular and mixed interstitial opacities	± Mild anemia; ± proteinuria
3 (severe)	General loss of condition or cachexia; fatigue with mild activity; frequent cough; ± dyspnea; ± right heart failure	Right ventricular and atrial enlargement; moderate-to-severe pulmonary artery enlargement; perivascular or diffuse mixed alveolar/interstitial opacities	Anemia; proteinuria
4 (very severe)	Caval syndrome; circulatory shock; icterus	Similar to above ± right heart failure (pleural effusion)	Anemia (hemolytic) ± thrombocytopenia; azotemia; elevated liver enzymes; hemoglobinuria

Modified from Nelson RW, Couto CG, eds: *Small animal internal medicine,* St Louis, 1998, Mosby.

Box 10-3.   Recommendatiions for Melarsamine
(Immiticide) Adulticide Therapy

Before Initiating Treatment
Confirm diagnosis
Pretreatment evaluation and management
Determine severity (class) of disease (see Table 10-1)
Determine immiticide treatment regimen

Standard Treatment for Class 1 and Most Class 2 Dogs
Draw 2.5 mg/kg of immiticide into a syringe, attach a fresh 23-
gauge needle: 1 inch for for dogs < 10 kg or 1.5 inch for dogs
> 10 kg
Administer by deep muscular injection to the epaxial muscles in
the L3–L5 region; avoid SQ leakage
Repeat steps 1 and 2 in 24 hours; use opposite side for injection
Enforced rest for 4–6 weeks minimum

Alternate Treatment for Class 3 and Some Class 2 Dogs
Symptomatic treatment as needed; enforced rest
When stable, administer one dose as described earlier in the
standard protocol
Continue symptomatic treatment and enforced rest
One month later, proceed with standard treatment as above

Modified from Nelson RW, Couto CG, eds: *Small animal internal medicine*,
St Louis, 1998, Mosby.

to the medications (toxicity, local tissue damage) or to
the infection itself (thromboembolic pulmonary disease, anaphylaxis from dying worms). Patients with

Box 10-4. Recommendations for Thiacetarsamide
(Caparsolate) Adulticide Therapy

Before Initiating Treatment
Confirm diagnosis
Pretreatment evaluation
Manage concurrent problems

Initial Thiacetarsamide Dose
Feed 30–60 minutes before treatment
Clip and prepare vein
Prepare syringe with thiacetarsamide dose (2.2 mg/kg) and
    syringe with saline flush
Insert butterfly needle into vein; if unsuccessful on first attempt,
    use another vein
Flush with saline to confirm venipuncture
Carefully inject thiacetarsamide, followed by saline flush
Remove needle and apply small pressure wrap to *avoid*
    hematoma

For Remaining Injections
Observe for vomiting, lethargy or depression, inappetence,
    fever, icterus, dehydration and bilirubinuria; if any of these
    symptoms are present, therapy may need to be discontinued
Examine previous venipuncture site; choose a different site for
    the next injection
Prepare and inject as for initial dose (steps 2–7)
A total of four injections are given 12 hours apart.

Modified from Nelson RW, Couto CG, eds: *Small animal internal medicine,*
St Louis, 1998, Mosby.

known thromboembolic disease, proteinuria, or pulmonary granulomas may be best managed by treating or controlling the complications before adulticide therapy. Currently, melarsamine is the recommended adulticide. Melarsamine is more efficacious and may be associated with fewer side effects than caparsolate.

Routine aspirin theraphy is no longer recommended in Heartworm disease because of the lack of beneficial antithrombotic effect. Heparin theraphy may be appropriate in some patients with severe pulmonary thrombosis.

PREVENTIVE TREATMENT Ivermectin (Heartguard 30) and Milbemycin oxime (Interceptor) are oral preparations given once monthly for prevention of infection. Although these drugs block the maturation of heartworm larvae, they are not used to kill the adult worms. These preventives may also combine medications to control gastrointestinal parasites as well. Diethylcarbamazine (DEC) is an older, once-daily preventive that is uncommonly administered. It has a narrower therapeutic dosing range compared with the monthly medications, and has been associated with idiosyncratic toxic hepatopathy and microfilariae-death anaphylaxis.

Feline Heartworm Disease

The cause and pathophysiology of feline heartworm disease are identical to those for the dog. However, there are some species differences in clinical manifestations and management of heartworm disease in cats. Box 10-5 outlines some differences between cats and dogs.

TREATMENT Treatment is often directed at the secondary complications (e.g., allergic pneumonitis), waiting for the worms to die naturally. Feline heartworm prevention is now frequently administered in endemic areas.

Box 10-5. Feline Heartworm Clinical Contrasts to Canine Heartworm

---

Overall disease prevalence is less than for dogs in the same general region

More difficult to diagnose (antigen + antibody test +/− thoracic radiograph needed)

Heartworms have shorter survival (< 2 years)

Increased frequency of aberrant worm migration

Rare circulating microfilariae

Thromboembolic disease and vascular obstruction more likely (relative worm size)

Allergic pneumonitis is common

Adulticide therapy is unrewarding (high mortality)

From Nelson RW, Couto CG, eds: *Small animal internal medicine, ed 2,* St Louis, 1998, Mosby.

11

Systemic Hypertension

Definition

Abnormally elevated systolic (primarily) and diastolic arterial blood pressure is defined as systemic hypertension (SHT). As a general rule, normal arterial blood pressure for most dogs is 100/65 to 160/100 mm Hg (systolic/diastolic), whereas 110/70 to 180/110 mm Hg is considered normal for cats and sighthound breeds of dogs.

Cause

Arterial blood pressure (BP) is the product of cardiac output (CO) and total peripheral vascular resistance

(TPR), that is BP = CO × TPR. In addition, CO is controlled by heart rate (HR) and stroke volume (SV) such that CO = HR × SV. Thus factors that cause an increase in vascular volume or TPR often lead to elevations in systemic blood pressure. Box 11-1 lists conditions associated with systemic hypertension.

Pathophysiology

The five basic mechanisms of systemic hypertension are in Box 11-2.

Box 11-1.   Conditions Associated with Systemic Hypertension

Renal disease[*]
Hyperthyroidism
Hyperadrenocorticism
Diabetes mellitus
Hypothyroidism
Acromegaly
Pheochromocytoma
Hyperaldosteronism
Hyperkinetic heart and anemia
Intracranial disease
Drugs (e.g., phenylpropanolamine)

[*]The most common cause in veterinary patients.

Box 11-2. Five Basic Pathophysiologic Mechanisms of Systemic Hypertension

1. Renal sodium retention
2. Sympathetic nervous system reactivity
3. Renin-angiotensin-aldosterone system (and AT II)
4. Endothelial cell dysfunction
5. Vascular hypertrophy

SHT tends to be a self-perpetuating process because many mechanisms overlap and antagonize others, particularly with chronicity. For example, renal disease may be associated with impaired sodium and water excretion, and elevations in renin-angiotensin-aldosterone system (RAAS). These factors contribute to the elevated arterial pressure by increasing vascular volume and promoting vasoconstriction (angiotensin [AT] II). Glomerular hypertension further injures the nephron, causing more renal compromise. Additional renal damage leads to greater impairment of sodium and water excretion, and exacerbations of RAAS (and TPR). It has also been proposed that AT II stimulates vascular endothelial hypertrophy and remodeling, perpetuating TPR in chronic disease. The fact that there are several intertwined pathophysiologies in SHT is likely responsible for need of multiple strategies to normalize blood pressure in some patients.

Presentation

Patients may present with a number of symptoms secondary to complications from SHT (Box 11-3). Certain organs are particularly sensitive to the vascular alterations of SHT and are referred to as *target organs*. These organs are the eye, kidney, heart, and brain. Some patients are screened or diagnosed with SHT based on finding a predisposing condition, even when complications from SHT are absent.

Diagnosis

Measuring elevated systolic blood pressure in a patient with reported complications or a predisposing con-

---

Box 11-3.   Complications of Systemic Hypertension

Blindness, retinal detachment or serous exudates
Hyphema
Glaucoma
Cerebral bleeding (e.g., circling, ataxia)
Epistaxis
Seizures
Nephrosclerosis (deterioration of renal function)
Left ventricular hypertrophy +/– outflow murmur
Syncope (arrhythmias)

dition is used to make the diagnosis of SHT (see Chapter 3).

Treatment

Patients with mild SHT and no clinical symptoms may not need antihypertensive therapy. These pets should be screened for an underlying condition and monitored frequently. Several strategies are often needed in treating moderate-to-severe SHT. Renal disease diets (low sodium, low protein) are helpful if renal dysfunction is known or suspected as a cause of SHT. Primary salt sensitivity is rare in small animals; thus diuretic therapy is of limited value and uncommonly prescribed. There are several drugs that may be chosen for initial control of SHT (Box 11-4). One medication at a time is administered, and the patient is reexamined every 1 to 2 weeks. It may take up to 2 weeks to see maximal results. Medications may be chosen based on the suspected pathophysiologic mechanism; however, clinician experience and preference often dictate drug choices.

Monitoring and Prognosis

Blood pressure should be reevaluated every 1 to 2 weeks until normalized. Monitoring pressure every 2 to 4 months may be sufficient in chronic, well-managed cases. Medications often need to be adjusted, supplemented, or replaced over time. The underlying condition may dictate more frequent monitoring. The prognosis for SHT varies and is closely correlated to the associated disease state.

Box 11-4. Common Antihypertensive Therapies

ACEis
Benazepril 0.25–0.5 mg/kg q24h PO (dog and cat)
Enalapril 0.25–0.5 mg/kg q12–24h PO (dog and cat)
Lisinopril 0.25–0.5 mg/kg q24h PO (dog)

Beta Blockers
Atenolol 0.2–1.0 mg/kg q12–24h PO (dog); 6.25–12.5 mg q12–24h PO (cat)
Esmolol 200–500 µg/kg IV over 1 minute; 25–200 µg/kg/min CRI (dog and cat)

Calcium Channel Blocker (Arterial Selective)
Amlodipine besylate 0.1–0.2 mg/kg q24h PO (dog); 0.625–1.25 mg q24h PO (cat)

Direct Vasodilator
Hydralazine 0.5–2 mg/kg q12h PO (dog and cat)

Nitric Oxide Donor
Nitroprusside 0.5–1 µg/kg/min CRI for hypertensive crisis (dog and cat)

ACEis, Angiotensin-converting enzyme inhibitors; *CRI*, constant rate infusion.

12

Common Cardiac Arrhythmias

General Considerations

Sinus rhythm is the normal cardiac rhythm that originates from the pacemaker (sinus node). Sinus rhythm is manifest by P-QRS-T, as described in Chapter 3. This rhythm is typically a regular rhythm; however, sinus arrhythmia is commonly observed in dogs as a normal finding (Figure 12-1). Sinus arrhythmia is characterized by normal P-QRS-T complexes that cyclically speed up and slow down, varying the heart rate and regularity. This rhythm is often associated with respirations and fluctuations of vagal tone during the respiratory cycle. The sinus pacemaker activity can also be described as

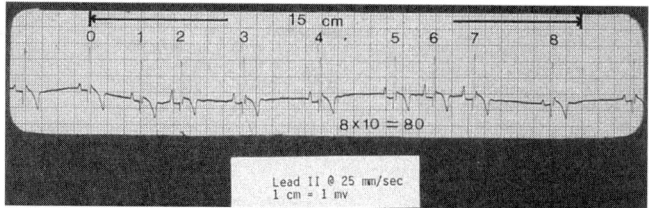

Figure 12-1.   Lead II at 25-mm/sec paper speed. An example of normal sinus arrhythmia in the dog. Note the regular irregularity of the R-R intervals. Fifteen centimeters or 30 large boxes at 25 mm/sec = 6 seconds; therefore the heart rate is approximately 80 beats/min.

"abnormally" slow (sinus bradycardia) or fast (sinus tachycardia) due to physiologic processes.

Ectopic Complexes

Ectopic complexes are abnormal impulses originating from outside the sinus node. These impulses often create an irregularity in the heart rhythm (pathologic arrhythmia). If these complexes are occurring consistently, there may also be abnormalities of heart rate (too fast or too slow). Ectopic complexes are described based on their origin (supraventricular versus ventricular) and their timing (premature or late/ escape) in relation to the previous QRS (Figure 12-2). Patients may or may not be symptomatic because of the arrhythmia. If symptoms are present, they are commonly associated with

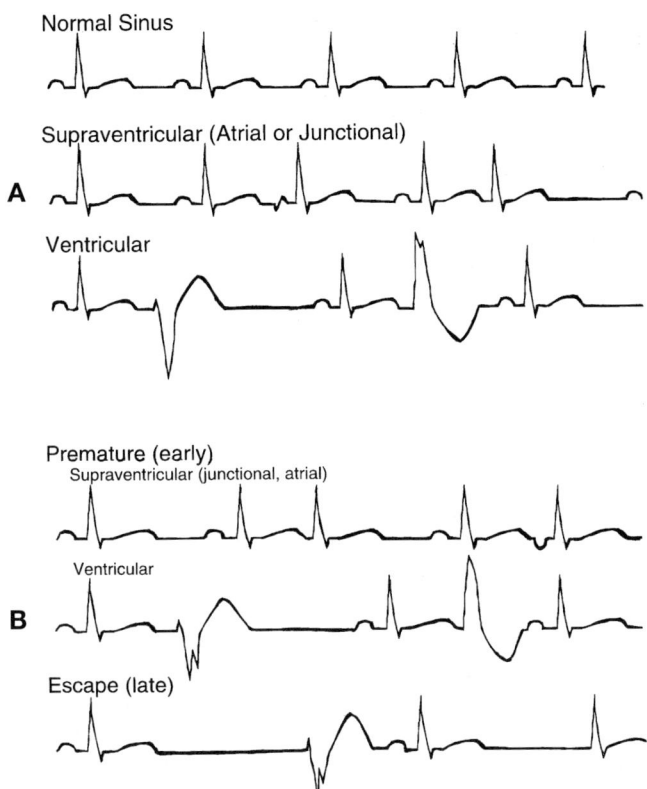

Figure 12-2. Diagrams illustrating the origin **(A)** and timing **(B)** of ectopic complexes. (*From Nelson RW, Couto CG, eds: Small animal medicine, ed 2, St Louis, 1998, Mosby.*)

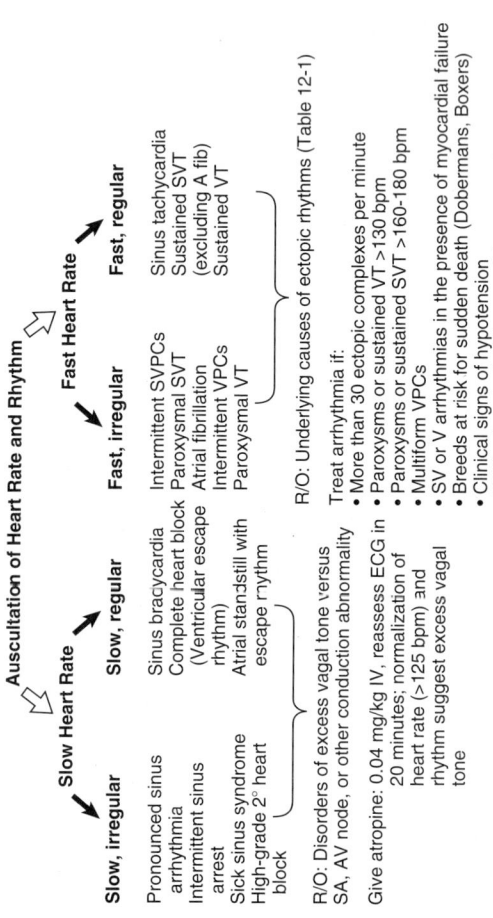

Auscultation of Heart Rate and Rhythm

Slow Heart Rate

Fast Heart Rate

Slow, irregular

Pronounced sinus arrhythmia
Intermittent sinus arrest
Sick sinus syndrome
High-grade 2° heart block

Slow, regular

Sinus bracycardia
Complete heart block (Ventricular escape rhythm)
Atrial standstill with escape rhythm

Fast, irregular

Intermittent SVPCs
Paroxysmal SVT
Atrial fibrillation
Intermittent VPCs
Paroxysmal VT

Fast, regular

Sinus tachycardia
Sustained SVT (excluding A fib)
Sustained VT

R/O: Disorders of excess vagal tone versus SA, AV node, or other conduction abnormality

Give atropine: 0.04 mg/kg IV, reassess ECG in 20 minutes; normalization of heart rate (>125 bpm) and rhythm suggest excess vagal tone

R/O: Underlying causes of ectopic rhythms (Table 12-1)

Treat arrhythmia if:
• More than 30 ectopic complexes per minute
• Paroxysms or sustained VT >130 bpm
• Paroxysms or sustained SVT >160-180 bpm
• Multiform VPCs
• SV or V arrhythmias in the presence of myocardial failure
• Breeds at risk for sudden death (Dobermans, Boxers)
• Clinical signs of hypotension
• VPCs close to the T wave of the proceeding complex (R-on-T phenomenon)

Figure 12-3. An algorithm for differential cardiac rhythm diagnoses by auscultation. *SVPC,* Supraventricular premature complex; *SVT,* supraventricular tachycardia; *VPC,* ventricular premature complex; *VT,* ventricular tachycardia.

Table 12-1. The Classic Four Types of Antiarrhythmic Drugs

Class	Channel Effects	Examples	Use or Comments
IA	Sodium, block	Quinidine, procainamide	Supraventricular and ventricular rhythms; inexpensive
IB	Sodium, block	Lidocaine, mexiletine, tocainide	Ventricular rhythms; affinity for diseased or ischemic muscle tissue
IC	Sodium, block	Flecainide, propafenone	Markedly inhibits Na^{2+} channels; rarely used
II	Beta receptor, block	Atenolol, propanolol, metoprolol, sotalol	Supraventricular rhythms using the AV node (i.e., atrial fibrillation); some ventricular rhythms
III	K^+ repolarizing, block	Amiodarone, sotalol, bretylium	Broad-spectrum class, supraventricular and ventricular rhythms Miscellaneous drug class, multiple mechanisms noted (i.e., sotalol)
IV	Calcium, block	Diltiazem, verapamil	Supraventricular rhythms using the AV node (i.e., atrial fibrillation)

weakness or collapse from extreme bradycardia or tachycardia. Sometimes the pathologic arrhythmia is the first symptom of heart disease. The common causes of ectopic complexes are given in Box 12-1.

Examples of Common Arrhythmias

See Figures 12-4 through 12-7.

Box 12-1.   Common Underlying Causes of Ectopic Complexes

Irritation or inflammation of heart muscle
Primary heart muscle disease
Cardiac chamber dilation
Myocardial ischemia
Electrolyte and acid-base imbalance
Toxins or drugs
Alterations in sympathetic nervous system tone

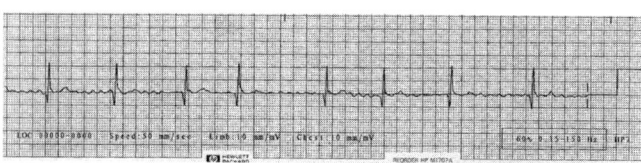

Figure 12-4.   Lead II. Atrial fibrillation in a Gorden Setter with DCM. Note the irregularly irregular R-R intervals and the bumpy baseline without identifiable P waves.

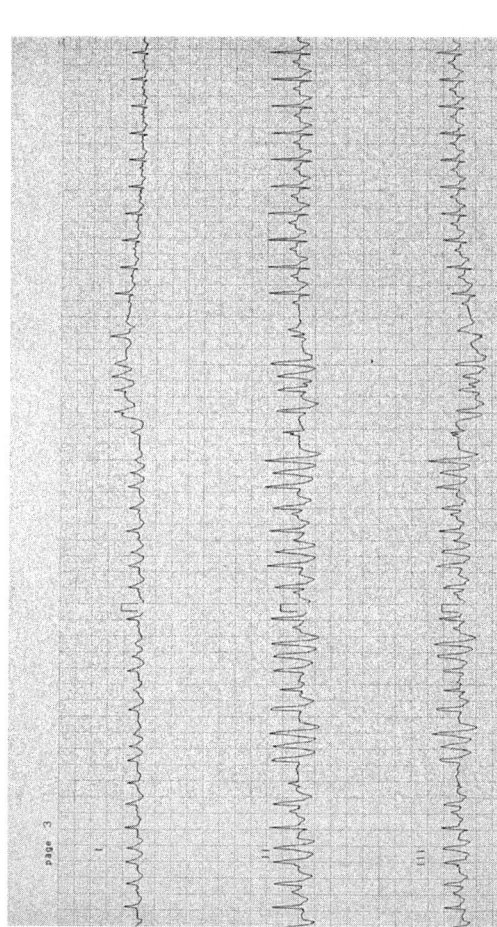

Figure 12-5. Leads I, II, and III at 25-mm/sec paper speed. Rapid paroxysmal ventricular tachycardia in a Boxer. This dog was given intravenous lidocaine and converted to normal sinus rhythm (last one third of strip).

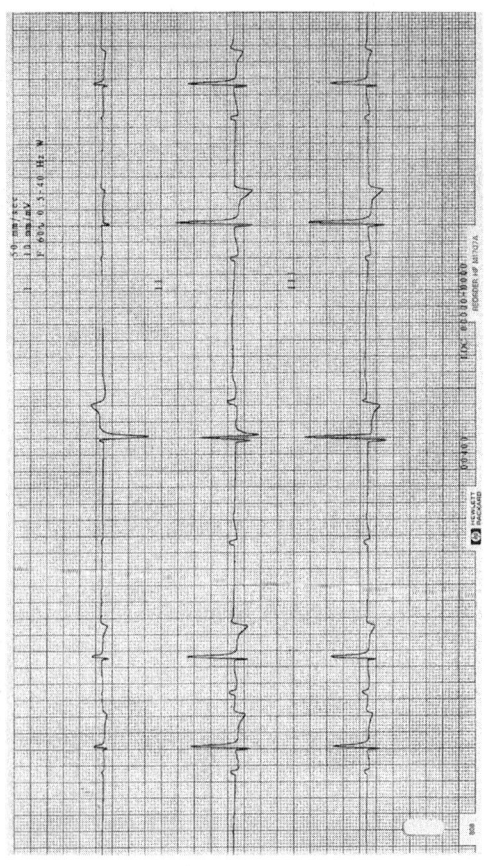

A

Figure 12-6. Leads I, II, and III at 50-mm/sec. An electrocardiogram obtained from a collapsing Cocker Spaniel with sinus bradycardia and first- and second-degree heart block before and after an atropine response test. **A,** Note the progressive P-R interval prolongation until the QRS is blocked. The third P wave is not followed by a QRS. The third QRS is a junctional escape beat (no P wave).

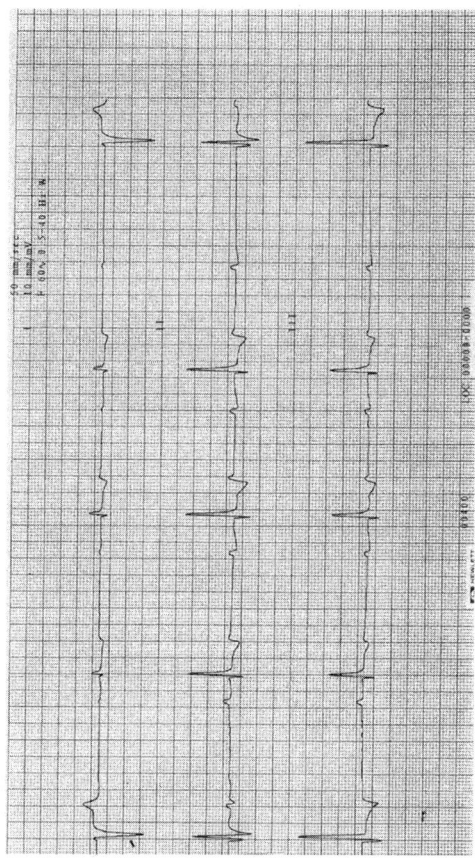

B

Figure 12-6.—cont'd. **B,** Note minimal response to atropine. The bradyarrhythmia is still present. This patient's bradycardia is not related to vagal tone, and thus a pacemaker is the treatment of choice.

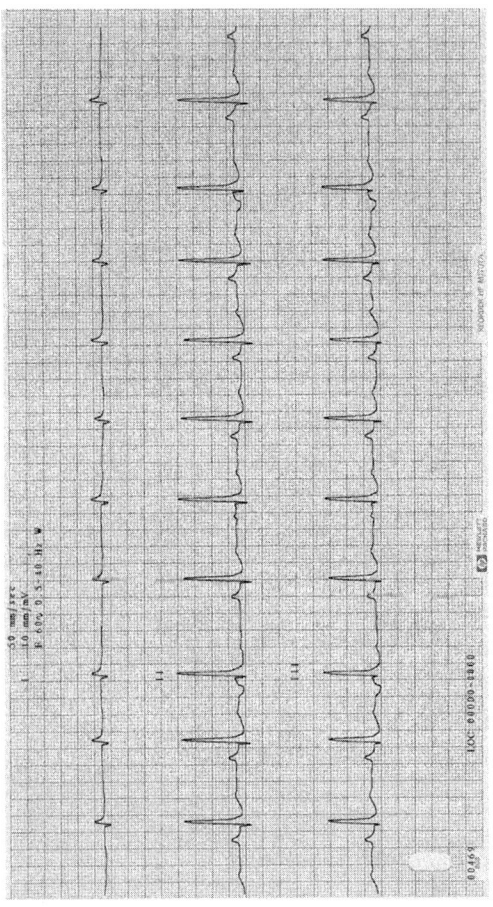

Figure 12-7. Leads I, II, and III at 25-mm/sec paper speed. Atrial premature contractions (complexes 3 and 9) in a dog with vegetative endocarditis. Note the negative P waves and prematurity of the R interval.

Appendix 1

Commonly Used Cardiovascular Drugs

Name (generic)	Drug Class	Actions	Indications	Dose	Side Effects
Acepromazine	Tranquilizer	Sedation	Anxiety, sedation Vasodilation	D: 0.03–0.1 mg/kg IV C: 0.03–0.2 mg/kg IM SQ	Hypotension Bradycardia
Amlodipine besylate	Vasodilator	Arteriodilation Selective Ca^{2+} blocker	Systemic hypertension Reduce afterload	D: 0.1–0.2 mg/kg q24h PO C: 0.625–1.25 mg/cat q24h PO C: ?	Hypotension
Amrinone	⊕ Inotrope	⊖ Phosphodiesterase Vasodilation Increased contractility	Systolic dysfunction DCM, poor CO Acute or critical CHF	D: 1–3 mg/kg IV D: 10–100 µg/kg/min CRI C: ?	Hypotension Gastrointestinal Arrhythmias
Atenolol	β_1-blocker	⊖ Inotrope ⊖ Chronotrope Prolongs AV conduction Slows SA recovery	SVT, some VT Diastolic dysfunction (i.e., HCM)	D: 0.2–1 mg/kg q12–24h PO (start low) C: 6.25–12.5 mg q12–24h PO	Bradycardia ⊖ Inotropic effect
Atropine	Anticholinergic	Vagolytic ⊕ chronotrope	Bradycardia Heart block	D: 0.02–0.04* mg/kg IV C: same	Tachycardia Hypotension Hypertension Gastrointestinal
Benazepril	ACE i	Vasodilation ↓ Aldosterone ↓ Vasopressin ↓ Norepinephrine	Volume overload CHF Systemic hypertension	D: 0.25–0.5 mg/kg q24h PO C: Same?	Hyperkalemia Hypotension Renal dysfunction Gastrointestinal
Buprenorphine	Tranquilizer Analgesic	Partial opiate agonist	Anxiety, sedation Analgesia	D: 0.0075–0.01 mg/kg IV C: not used	Hypotension Bradycardia ↓ respiration
Butorphanol	Tranquilizer Analgesic	Partial opiate agonist	Anxiety, sedation Analgesia Antitussive	D: 0.2–0.4 mg/kg IV, IM, SQ C: same Cough: 0.05–0.12 q8–2h PO	Excess sedation Slight bradycardia Gastrointestinal

Digoxin	⊕ Inotrope	↓Na+–K+ ATPase ↑ Na+–Ca2+ exchange Decreases SNS tone Normalizes baroreceptors Prolongs AV conduction	CHF, esp. systolic dysfunction Atrial fibrillation SVT	D: 0.005–0.01 mg/kg q12h C: 1/4 of 0.125-mg tab q3rd day PO ALWAYS start conservatively MONITOR serum levels	Gastrointestinal Anorexia Heart block Arrhythmias
Diltiazem	Ca2+ blocker Class IV	Ca2+ channel blocker Prolongs AV conduction Prolongs refractory times Less effect on SA node	Atrial fibrillation SVT Diastolic dysfunction (i.e., HCM)	D: 0.5–1.5 mg/kg q8h PO C: same or 15–30 mg q24h of extended release prep(Dilacor®)	Bradycardia Heart block Hypotension Gastrointestinal
Dobutamine	⊕ Inotrope	β-adrenergic stimulation (β₁ > β₂ > α)	Critical CHF, esp. w/o severe hypotension	D: 2–20 µg/kg/min CRI C: ? start low	Arrhythmias Hypertension
Dopamine	⊕ Inotrope Catecholamine	Releases cardiac NE Vasodilation (DA receptors— low dose) Vasoconstriction (α receptors—high dose)	Critical CHF Splanchnic vasodilation (lower doses) Circulatory shock	D: 2–10 µg/kg/min CRI C: same	Hypertension Tachyarrhythmias Gastrointestinal
Enalapril	ACEi	Vasodilation ↓ Aldosterone ↓Vasopressin ↓ Norepinephrine	Volume overload CHF Systemic hypertension	D: 0.25–1 mg/kg q12h PO C: 0.25–0.5 mg/kg q12–24h	Hypotension Hyperkalemia Renal dysfunction Gastrointestinal
Epinephrine	⊕ Inotrope Catecholamine	β-adrenergic stimulation (β₁ = β₂ > α) Vasoconstriction	Anaphylaxis CPR	D: 0.2 mg/kg IV or 0.1–1.0 µg/kg/min CRI C: same	Hypotension Arrhythmias Excitability Gastrointestinal

Continued

Name (generic)	Drug Class	Actions	Indications	Dose	Side Effects
Esmolol	β_1-blocker Class II	$\ominus$ Inotrope $\ominus$ Chronotrope Prolongs AV conduction Slows SA recovery time	SVT, some VT	D: 0.2–0.5 mg/kg slow IV or 0.025–0.2 mg/kg/ min CRI C: same ?	Bradycardia $\ominus$ Inotropic effect
Furosemide	Diuretic	↓ Na^+ resorption, ascending Loop of Henle K^+ excretion	CHF Volume overload	D: 1–3 mg/kg q8–12h PO or 2–5 mg/kg q4–6h IV, IM, SQ C: 1–2 mg/kg q12h, or 1–4 mg/kg q8–12h IV, IM, SQ	Dehydration Hypotension Electrolyte imbalance
Glycopyrrolate	Anticholinergic	Vagolytic $\oplus$ chronotrope	Bradycardia Heart block	D: 0.01–0.02 mg/kg IV, IM, SQ C: same	Tachycardia Hypertension Hypotension Gastrointestinal
Hydralazine	Vasodilator	Arterial dilation Direct action	Reduce afterload Systemic hypertension	D: 0.5–2 mg/kg q12h PO C: 2.5–5 mg q12h PO	Hypotension Tachycardia Fluid retention Gastrointestinal
Hydrochlorothiazide	Thiazide diuretic	↓ Na^+, Cl^- resorption, distal tubules	CHF; combine with Loop diuretic in diuretic resistance	D: 2–4 mg/kg q12h PO C: 1–2 mg/kg q12h PO	Dehydration Hypotension Hypokalemia
Isosorbide dinitrate	Vasodilator Nitrate	Venous > arterial Formation of NO	CHF	D: 0.5–2 mg/kg q8h PO C: ?	Hypotension Tachycardia Tolerance
Lisinopril	ACEi	Vasodilation ↓ Aldosterone ↓ Vasopressin ↓ Norepinephrine	Volume overload CHF Systemic hypertension	D: 0.25–0.5 mg/kg q24h PO C: same?	Hypotension Hyperkalemia Renal dysfunction Gastrointestinal

Drug	Class	Mechanism	Indication	Dose	Side effects
Lidocaine	Antiarrhythmic Class IB	Blocks Na$^+$ channel (esp. inactive state)	Ventricular arrhythmia esp. ischemic	D: 2–8 mg/kg slow IV or 25–80 µg/kg/min CRI C: 0.25–0.5 mg/kg slow IV or 10–20 µg/kg/min CRI	Drowsiness Depression Seizures (esp. cats) Gastrointestinal
Metoprolol	β$_1$-blocker Class II	⊖ Inotrope ⊖ Chronotrope Prolongs AV conduction Slows SA recovery time	SVT, some VT	D: 0.2–1 mg/kg q8h PO C: ?	Bradycardia ⊖ Inotropic effect
Mexiletine	Antiarrhythmic Class IB	Blocks Na$^+$ channel (esp. inactive state)	Ventricular arrhythmia	D: 4–10 mg/kg q8h PO C: not used	Gastrointestinal Depression Seizures
Nitroglycerin (ointment, 2%)	Vasodilator Nitrate	Venous > arterial Formation of NO	CHF	D: 1/2–1 inch q4–6h cutaneously C: 1/4–1/2 inch q4–6h	Hypotension Tachycardia Tolerance
Nitroprusside	Vasodilator	NO donor	Hypertensive crisis	D: 0.5–15 µg/kg/min CRI C: same	Hypotension Gastrointestinal Cyanide toxicity
Procainamide	Antiarrhythmic Class IA	Blocks Na$^+$ channel Prolongs atrial and ventricular refractory time	Supraventricular and ventricular arrhythmia	D: 6–20 mg/kg IV, IM, PO or 10–20 µg/kg/min CRI C: 1–2 mg/kg slow IV or 10–20 µg/kg/min CRI; 6–20 mg/kg q8h IM	Hypotension Gastrointestinal Wide QRS Multiform VT

Continued

Name (generic)	Drug Class	Actions	Indications	Dose	Side Effects
Propantheline Br	Anticholinergic	Vagolytic $\oplus$ chronotrope	Bradycardia Heart block	D: 3.75–30 mg q8h PO C: ?	Tachycardia Hypertension Hypotension Gastrointestinal
Propranolol	β_1, β_2-blocker Class II	$\ominus$ Inotrope $\ominus$ Chronotrope Prolongs AV conduction Slows SA recovery time	SVT, some VT Diastolic dysfunction (i.e., HCM)	D: 0.1–1 mg/kg q8h PO; 0.02–0.1 g/kg slow IV C: 2.5–10 mg/cat q8h; IV same	Bradycardia $\ominus$ Inotropic effect Bronchoconstriction
Quinidine	Antiarrhythmic Class IA	Bronchoconstriction Blocks Na$^+$ channel Prolongs atrial and ventricular refractory time Some anticholinergic	SVT and ventricular arrhythmia	D: 6–20 mg/kg q6–8h IV, IM, PO q8h PO	Hypotension Gastrointestinal Wide QRS AV block
Sotalol	Antiarrhythmic Class III	$\uparrow$ channel blocker β_1, β_2-blocker $\ominus$ Inotrope $\ominus$ Chronotrope Prolongs action potential	Refractory/malignant VTs and SVTs	D: 1–2 mg/kg q12h PO C: ?	Tachycardias Bradycardia $\ominus$ Inotropic effect Bronchoconstriction Multiform VT
Spironolactone	Diuretic K$^+$ sparing	Antagonizes aldosterone (distal renal tubule) Excrete Na$^+$, Cl$^-$ Conserves K$^+$	CHF, additive to other diuretic therapies	D: 2 mg/kg q12h PO C: 1 mg/kg q12h PO	Dehydration Hypotension Hyperkalemia Gastrointestinal

$\oplus$, Positive; $\ominus$, negative; α, alpha; *ACEi*, angiotensin-converting enzyme inhibitor; *AV*, atrioventricular; β, beta; *CHF*, congestive heart failure; *CO*, cardiac output; *CPR*, cardiopulmonary resuscitation; *CRI*, constant rate infusion; *DA*, dopamine receptors; *DCM*, dilated cardiomyopathy; *HCM*, hypertrophic cardiomyopathy; *NE*, norepinephrine; *NO*, nitric oxide; *SA*, sinoatrial; *SNS*, sympathetic nervous system; *SVT*, supraventricular tachycardia; *VT*, ventricular tachycardia. *Dose for drug challenge.

Appendix 2

Diagnostic Equipment Commonly Used in Cardiovascular Medicine

Equipment	Model or Type	Manufacturer
Blood Pressure Monitor		
Noninvasive blood pressure monitor (ultrasonic Doppler flow detector)	811-B	Parks Medical Electronics, Inc., Aloha, OR 1-800-547-6427
Noninvasive blood pressure monitor (Oscillometric method)	Dinamap Monitor 1846 SX/P Many models	Critikon, Tampa, FL
Blood pressure cuffs	Human pediatric Infant sizes	Parks Medical Electronics, Inc., Aloha, OR Critikon, Tampa, FL Zefon International, St. Petersburg, FL
Electrocardiograph		
Electrocardiograph, diagnostic	100/200 series	Hewlett Packard, McMinnville, OR
Electrocardiograph, diagnostic	Burdick E200–650 Series	Siemens/Burdick, Milton, WI
Electrocardiograph, diagnostic	MAC 500, 1200, 5000	Marquette, many retailers
Electrocardiograph, surgical monitoring	Many models	Many companies (above) offer surgical monitoring equipment, often combined with oscillometric blood pressure monitor

Suggested Readings

Birchard SJ, Sherding RG, eds: *Saunders' manual of small animal practice*, ed 2, Philadelphia, 2001, WB Saunders Company.

Bonagura JD, ed: *Kirk's current veterinary therapy XII*, Philadelphia, 1995, WB Saunders Company.

Bonagura JD, ed: *Kirk's current veterinary therapy XIII*, Philadelphia, 2000, WB Saunders Company.

Ettinger SJ, Feldman EC, eds: *Textbook of veterinary Internal medicine: diseases of the dog and cat*, ed 5, Philadelphia, 2001, WB Saunders Company.

Fox PR, Sisson D, Moise NS, eds: *Textbook of canine and feline cardiology*, ed 2, Philadelphia, 1999, WB Saunders Company.

Kittleson MD, Kienle RD, eds: *Small animal cardiovascular medicine*, St Louis, 1999, Mosby.

Morgan RV, ed: *Handbook of small animal practice*, ed 3, Philadelphia, 1997, WB Saunders Company.

Nelson RW, Couto CG, eds: *Small animal internal medicine*, ed 2, St Louis, 1998, Mosby

Tilley LP, Goodwin JK, eds: *Manual of canine and feline cardiology*, ed 3, Philadelphia, 2001, WB Saunders Company.

Tilley LP, Miller MS, Smith FWK: *Canine and feline cardiac arrhythmias*, Philadelphia, 1993, Lea & Febiger.

Index

Page numbers followed by "t" indicate tables; page numbers followed by "b" indicate boxes